STEVEN G. ALDANA, PhD

Culture Clash

How We Win The Battle For Better Health

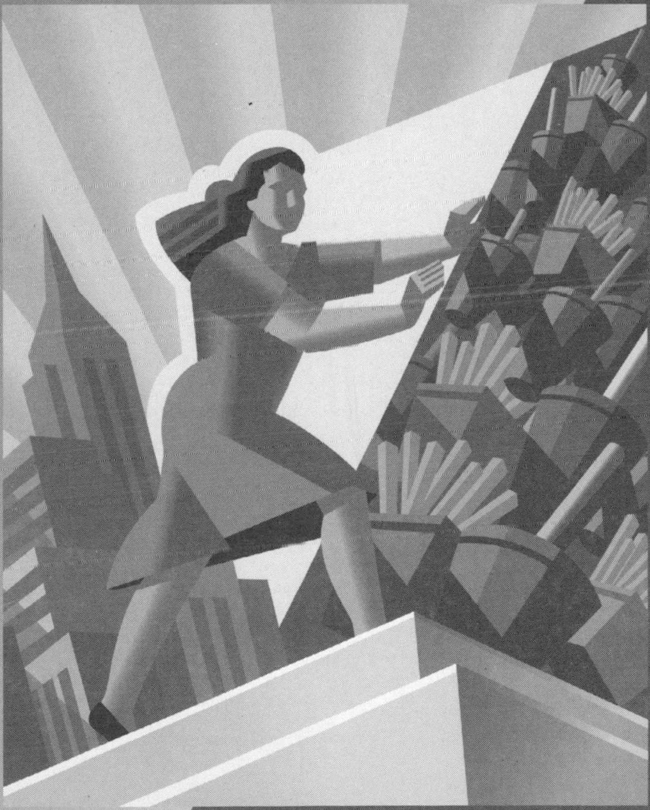

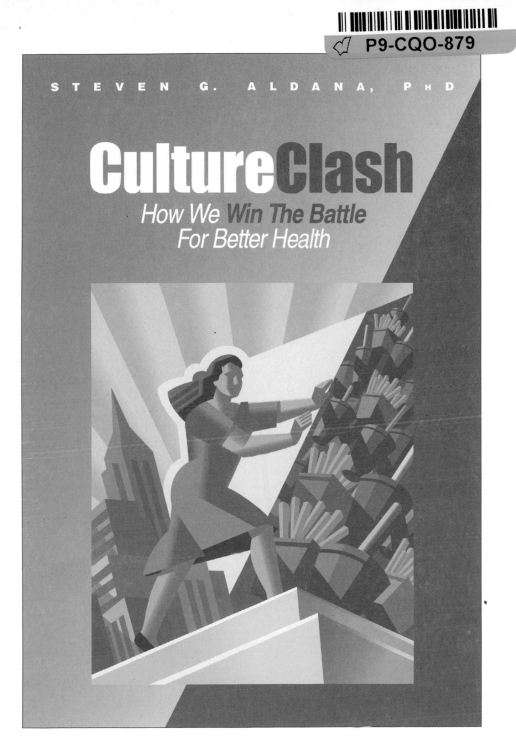

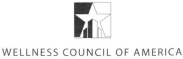

WELLNESS COUNCIL OF AMERICA

Library of Congress Catalog-in-Publication Data

Aldana, Steve G., 1962-
Culture Clash: How We Win The Battle For Better Health / Steven G. Aldana.
p. cm.
Includes bibliographical references and index.
Library of Congress Control Number: 2012921849
ISBN 978-0-9758828-8-7

1. Healthy living 2. Weight control. 3. Chronic disease prevention. I. Title.

RA776.9.A65 2013 613'.0979
QBI04-200466

Printed in the U.S.A.

Cover design by Leo Kundas.

Table Of Contents

Preface

BATTLING THICK, BLACK SMOKE RESIDENTS FROM CLEVELAND, OHIO USED SHOVELS AND PITCH FORKS TO TRY TO KEEP A FIRE FROM SPREADING THROUGH THE NEARBY FORESTS INTO HOMES AND BARNS. It seemed as though nothing could extinguish the fire. The year was 1868 and this was no ordinary fire. At the time, a large number of steel refineries and chemical companies were located along the Cuyahoga River which passes through the center of present day Cleveland, Ohio. There were few if any pollution controls and environmental regulations that could prevent industrial waste from being dumped into the surrounding rivers. The fire the residents were fighting was actually the Cuyahoga River, which had burst into flames. Years of dumping chemicals into the river had turned it into a flammable chemical concoction that only lacked a source of ignition. Not only was this practice legal, it was accepted waste management practice throughout the world. Between 1868 and 1969, the river caught fire ten times.

The fire that started in 1969 was the one that caught the attention of the world. Pictures published in national magazines showed the scorching flames rolling across the entire surface of the river. This last fire marked a turning point in the control and management of industrial waste. Residents and politicians finally looked into the problem and decided that significant changes needed to be made. Tired of the bad press and growing public discontent, businesses in Cleveland gave in to public and government pressure and began cleaning up. Today, the river has been dramatically rehabilitated. It even contains live fish and abundant wildlife.

For 100 years, no one seemed to care about the pollution in the river. No one seemed to mind that all the fish were dead or that local drinking water was contaminated with toxins. The only time people became concerned was when it burst into flames and even then, the worry abated once the fires were extinguished. Many of the residents worked in the plants and factories and their livelihood depended on the success of those businesses. Ignorance and greed were the biggest reasons the river was treated as a dump. Rather than spend money to properly dispose of chemical waste it was cheaper, faster and a lot easier to just dump it in the river. For decades, businesses fought any efforts to change their operations. Cleaning up the river and carefully disposing of industrial waste would be very expensive. These businesses provided jobs. They helped fuel the Industrial Revolution and were an important factor in expanding the U.S. economy. For 100 years, business owners exerted substantial influence over local and state politicians and with their combined financial and political power they were permitted to continue to dump waste into the river.

The whole story of the Cuyahoga River goes something like this:

- People don't see a problem with the polluted river.
- Businesses are very happy.

Time passes…
- People begin to think the pollution in the river may be a problem.
- Businesses are happy.

Time passes…
- More people think something should be done.
- Businesses refuse to admit there is a problem and vigorously resist change.
- Government doesn't want to hurt business, that's bad.

Time passes…
- The world sees pictures of a river burning and public opinions about pollution change.
- Businesses are forced to change their processes, the government fines violators, established waste disposal habits are changed and the river begins to heal.

The story of the life, death and subsequent rehabilitation of the Cuyahoga River provides an excellent metaphor for talking about your health. The parallels between the two issues are very similar.

The story of health for most people in western societies goes like this:

- Most people have unhealthy behaviors, but think they are healthy.
- Businesses are very happy.

Time passes…

- People slowly begin to discover unhealthy behaviors lead to elevated health risks and very poor health.
- Businesses are happy.

Time passes…

- More people than ever are obese or have chronic diseases, but find it extremely difficult to change behaviors.

Time passes…

- Businesses and government refuse to admit there is a problem or don't have the political will to change. Government doesn't want to hurt business or jobs, that's bad.
- Many people of the world have more body fat and diabetes than any other time in world history.

Time is still passing…

Unlike the Cuyahoga River there isn't an ending to this story yet, it's still being written. Personal health for most people is still on a steady, downward trend. The business and political forces in our society are either unwilling or unable to do much to alter the forces in our lives that cause us to have unhealthy behaviors.

As the Cuyahoga River became increasingly more polluted it caught fire at least 10 times over a 100-year period. The fires were just symptoms of a much bigger problem: a well-established business culture and tradition of using the river as a waste dump. Like the river, our society and culture shows symptoms of poor public health that catch the public's attention, but these symptoms are almost never linked back to the true source of the problem: a powerful and well-established culture of unhealthy living.

The symptoms of poor health I'm talking about are not as dramatic as a burning river, but they do act as warnings that something is very wrong. The amount of physical activity adults get has not changed much despite national efforts to increase physical activity. Our diets have changed dramatically, with highly processed foods now being the staple of most diets. Among children born in the year 2000, between 30 and 50% will be diabetic before they reach age 50.[1] Over 67% of all adults in the U.S. are now overweight or obese. We have more diabetes and body fat than at any other time in world history and over 70% of the $2.5 trillion Americans spend on health care every year is from preventable chronic diseases.

To some, the worsening trends in poor health suggest that something about the way we live our lives has changed. Almost everyone has the suspicion that it wasn't always this way. It seems there are a lot more overweight people around these days. A lot more people suffer from diabetes and just about everyone over 50 takes some form of medication to help lower health risks. Children seem to be fatter than they used to be. There is strong scientific evidence that suggests that these suspicions are correct.

Despite the symptoms of poor health and an unhealthy culture that we now see, not everyone agrees that there is anything wrong with the way we live our lives. Some businesses and organizations proclaim that poor health is nothing but a myth, perpetuated by an overreaching government and scientists wanting more money for research. (**www.consumerfreedom.com**) These groups claim there is nothing to fix, because nothing is broken. They point out that people of western civilizations live longer than ever so what could possibly be wrong with the way we live our lives? These naysayers are banding together, creating political action groups, lobbying organizations, and collectively funding national marketing campaigns to convince the public and the politicians that there is absolutely nothing wrong with our foods.

In most cases, these naysayers profit financially from the current situation and have a vested interest in seeing that nothing changes. The combined business and political efforts of industry are working in direct conflict with your efforts to have a long, healthy life. Let me restate that in a slightly different way: your extra body fat, your high blood pressure, your diabetes, your cancer, your heart disease, your high blood cholesterol, your erectile dysfunction…the list goes on, are a direct result of business, government and society. I realize these are pretty strong words.

Industry, society, culture, government, tradition and even capitalism are all responsible for creating the culture we live in. It's you and your desires for good health vs. the culture we live in and so far you're getting your butt kicked. You may not be willing to admit it, but you are a product of this unhealthy culture and your health is directly impacted by those who care more about money than your health.

It's not just Americans who are gaining weight; it's the citizens of every westernized country in the world. We're all failing to reach and maintain a healthy body weight because almost everything in our culture is working against us. From a societal and cultural perspective the cards are clearly stacked against you.

Identifying The Problem

I've spent my entire adult life working to help people have optimal health and a long, high quality life. I've published over 100 articles, research papers and books on the ability of healthy behaviors to prevent, arrest and in some cases reverse chronic diseases. The scientists I work with and others around the world have been thinking, studying and experimenting with ways to help people adopt and maintain healthy behaviors. Yet, in the past 50 years, the health of Americans and other westernized countries has steadily gotten worse. I fear that most of us are like the early residents of Cleveland who didn't like the river catching on fire, but weren't quite sure what to do about it. Many of them were upset with how the fires affected their homes and livelihoods, but they may have felt powerless to confront big business and politicians. Worse, I'm afraid that most people don't know what the real problem is.

Scientists and society have suggested lots of explanations for the cause of our continued health decline. Bad genes are easy to blame. They make the perfect scapegoat. "My father has high blood pressure, my mother has high blood pressure and now I have high blood pressure. I must have the gene. I place full blame for my poor health on the genes I inherited from my parents." "My mom and dad are both fat and I'm fat so I must have the same fat genes." "You skinny people are lucky. You have parents who are skinny too." Maybe your poor health can be blamed on your genes, but not likely. It's more likely you have the same health behaviors as your parents because you all live in exactly the same culture and environment and have the same eating and exercise habits. Genes can influence the diseases we get, but these cases are very rare. Compared to unhealthy lifestyles, genes have a very small impact on our health.

No one likes to feel guilty or weak. When we finger genetics as the problem, we can remove any guilt we may have for our poor behaviors. Rather than suffer from the knowledge that "I've" been making poor choices, we can blame our genes for our poor health. It places the blame on something we have no control over, a bunch of twisted cellular proteins we received from mom and dad. "It's not my fault, it's my genes." But this explanation for our poor health is incorrect. Seventy to 90% of our chronic diseases are caused by lifestyle choices, not genetics.[2]

So, if it's not genetics, what is the real cause of our continued decline in health? Is it our high fat diet? How about soda? Perhaps we can blame the school lunch program for making our kids fat? The Internet and video games have made us more sedentary—can we blame the World Wide Web? Fast food is everywhere now; surely fast food must be the problem. Maybe it's the health care industry. They make lots of money treating sick people. Pesticides and herbicides are in our food, perhaps the chemicals we've added to our foods are making us sick?

Bacon! It must be bacon, nothing that tastes that good can be good for you and we eat a lot of bacon. I was giving a talk in Wisconsin a few years ago and I drove past a billboard for a regional hamburger restaurant called Carvers. The billboard used just two things to make a compelling message to the public. The marketing staff at Carvers put a picture of a chocolate milk shake and a plate of bacon on a giant billboard with the words: Shakes and Bacon. Brilliant, it was almost enough to get me to pull off the freeway at the next exit, but I didn't. A diet of shakes and bacon is not likely to result in optimal health.

It has taken many, many years of research and critical thought to figure out why our health has gotten steadily worse. I'm proud to say that we know the cause and I'm even prouder to say we have the solution. Despite what the critics, politicians, industry and even some of our own scientists may say, it is the only long-term solution. I can hear what you are thinking, "Yeah right, that's a pretty bold declaration, what makes you think you are so right?" "Who is to say someone else won't write another book that claims to have 'the' solution?" These are fair questions and I promise to address each of them in detail, but first you should know that I'm the biggest skeptic I know. My scientific training causes me to question everything. I don't come to any conclusions lightly. I need evidence, real world examples, a carefully developed rationale, and lots and lots of supportive proof before I'll seriously consider an issue. Once I like the idea, I'll let it sit for a while. I let it stew around in my brain while I think about every possible error in my thinking. I'll bring it up with colleagues and other respected thinkers in my field. We'll debate, argue and challenge every notion.

The mystery we have solved is this: How come so many people are experiencing chronic diseases and gaining excessive body weight and what is a realistic, long-term solution that anyone can use to get healthier? The title of this book, Culture Clash, gives you a clue to the reasons why so many struggle to have good health. Once we understand the cause, we can begin to identify the real solutions. I want you to see the same information I've been seeing and studying. Think of your poor health as a mystery and we are about to start examining all the clues and puzzle pieces that lead to the only realistic solution.

We'll start by talking about the problem—just how bad our health has become. The first section of the book will show you the most recent symptoms that prove that most of us are losing the battle for good health. Then, to see how we've gotten to this point we're going to turn back the clock and watch it all happen again. We're going to learn how we have slowly, but dramatically changed our way of living. We'll talk about how our culture has changed, how the food industry has carefully engineered foods to maximize their addictive properties and how our modern civilization has altered the food we eat and our exercise patterns.

After these initial chapters, the solution to the mystery will be revealed. You may not like the solution because it's not easy. It's not a pill or quick fix. It's going to take some effort on your part. Think about all the people you know who have healthy behaviors. You know people who eat healthy, exercise regularly and have a healthy body weight. They live in the same geographic location that you do. They may shop at the same stores and pass the same billboards. You may both work at the same workplace. Despite all the pressures to eat unhealthy foods, they have somehow been able to rise above the cultural fray. They are successful at surrounding themselves with people, foods, priorities and strategies that allow them to live a healthy lifestyle even when the odds of doing so are overwhelmingly stacked against them. They have figured out a way to maintain a healthy body weight and avoid the chronic diseases that most people struggle with. Many people you know have already recognized the solution.

We've Been Here Before

There are many examples of how our society has gradually gone down an unsustainable path, noticed the error of our ways and changed. The history of the Cuyahoga River is a perfect example that shows us that despite how bad things can become, change is possible. It may take time, lots of it, but with the correct amount of influence in just the right places, it is possible for societies to make dramatic cultural course corrections. After 100 years of pollution, critical media exposure and increased environmental awareness, industries in Cleveland, Ohio decided that the price of making changes was less than the price of maintaining the status quo. Public opinion had turned and the clean-up process had begun. A new culture of environmentally friendly manufacturing was initiated. Though the polluters resisted the change, the cost of not changing would have been too burdensome.

Another similar cultural change has occurred in the U.S. In the early 1940s Los Angeles, California was experiencing air pollution so bad that visibility was reduced to three blocks. The four million residents in Los Angeles were suffering from respiratory discomfort, nausea, vomiting and smarting eyes. It was finally determined that automobiles and heavy industry were to blame, but like Cleveland, business was good and jobs were plentiful. California was booming. It wasn't until the citizens started pressuring government and businesses that any changes were implemented. It took over 50 years, but today, California has the strictest air quality regulations in the world and they also have some of the best air quality. They had created an unhealthy environment that was literally killing people and were still able to make a dramatic course correction.

At one point, almost half of all Americans were smokers. Cigarette smoking was encouraged by doctors, government and especially business. The culture of tobacco use was the norm. Smoking was permitted everywhere. It's hard to imagine, but at one time it was legal to smoke on airplanes. Then, research starting appearing that showed the harmful effects of tobacco. Big Tobacco challenged the research and hired big law firms to fight anyone who tried to stop them. These legal battles raged on for decades, and in fact they are still ongoing. States sued to recover the costs they were paying to treat tobacco related illnesses. Individuals sued, Canada sued, and the federal government sued Big Tobacco. The media jumped on board with more research results and local and state governments started implementing non-smoking policies and rules. Just like the polluters of the Cuyahoga River, Big Tobacco fought for decades to maintain the status quo. They have spent enormous amounts of money fighting all who oppose them. Yet, despite the fear of taking on the establishment by those who think Big Tobacco is wrong to produce a product that causes death, cultural changes are occurring. Today 22% of Americans smoke.

Just like farmers in Brazil, India and Africa, there are around 5,000 farmers in the U.S. who still grow tobacco. Every day they work in the fields growing, tending and harvesting the tobacco leaves used to produce cigarettes. Their daily efforts produce a product that kills five million people every year. Despite the evidence against tobacco use, they do it for one reason…the money. Clearly, having 22% of the U.S. population still smoking is unacceptable, but that is way better than 50%. This is like cleaning the Cuyahoga to keep it from catching fire, but still dumping enough pollutants to poison the water and kill all the local wildlife.

Admittedly, the poor health we are experiencing is not as simple as businesses selling products that are not good for us. After all, we as consumers have the option of picking where we want to spend our dollars and how we want to live our lives. It is ultimately our choice to smoke or eat lots of shakes and bacon. However, if the environment you live in makes it difficult or even impossible to make healthy choices than your freedom to choose has been greatly restricted. Your freedom to make healthy choices has been taken away. That is precisely the position where Americans and members of all western societies find themselves—stuck in a culture and environment where healthy behaviors are difficult to make.

The Battle Begins

Some have considered this to be a David vs. Goliath battle. We want to have good health and a long life while technology, business, government, tradition, culture and human nature work against us. It is an uphill battle, but a battle that can and is being won. If I didn't think this battle could be won I never would have quit my job. For 20 years I worked as a full, tenured professor at several universities. Tenure is a strange academic rule that says once you reach tenure status, you can never lose your job without just cause. It's as close to lifelong job security as you can get. After 20 years of studying and researching the causes of poor health and seeing firsthand how individuals could transform their lives I realized that my ability to impact health would always be greatly limited if I stayed in academia. I talked it over with my wife and decided to leave my cushy, well-paid professorship. The evidence for the worsening of health was everywhere and it was only going to get worse. That was six years ago. Today, the struggle for good health has only intensified. Right now the lines are being drawn and just like the battle to save the Cuyahoga River, the battle to have better health has begun.

PART I

Why Should I Care?

CHAPTER 1

White Smoke

AS A YOUNG BOY I HAD A KNACK FOR TAKING THINGS APART, BUT NOT BEING ABLE TO PUT THEM BACK TOGETHER AGAIN. MY PARENTS USUALLY LET ME DO THIS BECAUSE THE THINGS I TOOK APART WERE USUALLY ALREADY BROKEN. I had an eight track player, microwave, television, lawn mower engine and other things torn apart in a big box in the garage. In the beginning I couldn't put them back together, let alone fix them, but I was learning how things worked. After a while I got to be really good at fixing things. That may well be the main reason my wife married me. Soon, neighbors found out I could fix things and ever since I've been helping my family and neighbors fix stuff.

One day a neighbor asked if I would take a look at his car. He pulled into the drive way and revved the engine. White smoke came pouring out of the tail pipe. It was moist, slightly sweet smelling and did not smell like burning oil. I had a pretty good idea what the problem was before he even had time to explain some of the car's symptoms. I asked him if his check engine light had come on in the recent past. He said that it had, but he got tired of seeing it and had placed a small piece of black electrical tape over the light. With the tape blocking the check engine light, he could ignore the warning and be on his merry way, as though there was nothing to worry about. White smoke in the tail pipe usually means one of two things: a blown head gasket or a cracked engine. Regardless, the engine will soon stop running and the cost to fix either one is high (thousands of dollars). I soon discovered that my neighbor had a very slow radiator leak. He let the problem continue until his engine got so hot that it blew a head gasket. His car was toast.

Through my experience with cars and fixing stuff I had learned to recognize symptoms and signs of wear and tear. In the case of my neighbor, neglecting the early signs (a check engine light) ended up ruining his car. The white smoke he was so worried about was nothing more than a symptom of a much bigger, more painful problem—a blown head gasket.

Let's look at some more white smoke. This simple graph shows the percentage of adults who are clinically obese. It's pretty easy to understand. On the bottom it shows different years since 1961. The dots on the graph show the percentage of adults (people 20 years old and older) who are clinically obese. The trend starts at about 13% in 1961 and is currently at about 35%.

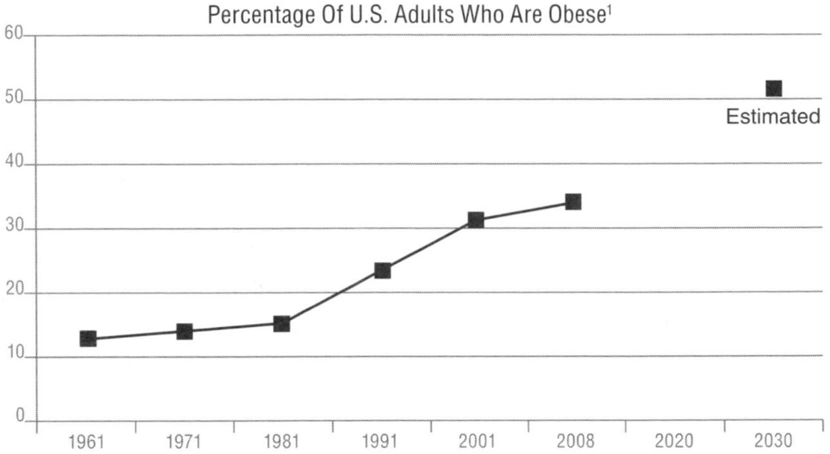

In this graph, obesity is determined from the Body Mass Index (BMI). You can determine your BMI using the table at the end of this chapter. The graph shows the percentage of adults who have BMI scores of 30 or greater. If your BMI is 30 or more you are considered obese.

Between 1961 and today the number of adults who are obese has increased 150%. The obesity trend for children and adolescents is worse. They have gotten fatter at an even faster rate. Scientists have looked carefully at this trend and have estimated that by the year 2030 over 51% of all adults will be obese.[2] This is shown in the graph as the black dot in the upper right. This estimate suggests that in the next few decades over half of adults will be clinically obese.

Not shown in the graph is the number of people who are overweight, but not obese. This number has increased as well. If we add up all the people who are overweight or obese we get 68% of all adults in the U.S. This is every adult with a BMI of 25 or greater. This is the highest prevalence of overweight ever recorded in the U.S., but next year it will likely be higher because as the graph shows, we get bigger every year.

Okay, the graph shows that we are fat and getting fatter and I'm sure that you already knew that before you started reading this book. Some of you are wondering if the rules for measuring obesity have changed. That's a great question because during this same time the rules for high blood pressure, high blood cholesterol and high blood glucose have all changed. The rules for these keep getting tighter. What used to be considered a healthy cholesterol level is now unhealthy and so the researchers keep lowering the value needed to be considered healthy. Researchers have been learning that what used to be considered healthy, may not be so—so they readjust the rules to agree with the current findings. They change the rules as more is learned. The rules for BMI have not changed. The definitions of overweight and obesity have been the same for 50 years. The chart is a consistent and accurate reflection of what has and is about to happen to us and our body weight.

This graph is exactly like the white smoke that was pouring out of my neighbor's car. It's a symptom or sign of something bigger. Other than the fact that my neighbor didn't particularly like to drive around town in a car that was putting out a smoke screen, the smoke wasn't a problem. The smoke didn't cause any problems. Yes, it was an inconvenience, and yes, people didn't like having smoke blown at them, but the smoke itself was nothing to be worried about. The symptoms or signs revealed by the chart show that we are getting bigger, much bigger, but is this a problem? Should we be concerned about our slow, gradual march toward greater body fat? All we need to do to make the trend toward obesity continue is to eat larger quantities of delicious foods, avoid exercise when possible, spend lots of time lying around watching television, sit in our cars and sit in front of our computers. Gaining body fat is not a problem, it's actually a pleasure. Weight gain is a side effect of our mostly pleasurable, socially acceptable eating behaviors.

The problem is not with the gaining of weight; the problem occurs when the extra weight starts to change our health and quality of life. The chart documents how our body fat is changing, but it reveals nothing about what really happens when we gain weight, nor does it tell us what the real problem is. It's just a warning sign.

Skinny People Are Not Exempt

If 68% of all adults are overweight or obese that leaves 32% of all adults who have a healthy body weight. I have a friend who is part of this group. She had recently gotten a physical from her doctor and had completed a blood draw to evaluate her blood glucose and cholesterol. She received a one page lab report in the mail showing her results. The report showed that she had a healthy body weight, but she doesn't get much exercise and her bad cholesterol (LDL) was high. Having a high LDL level increases her risk of cardiovascular disease. At that moment she was faced with a decision. She could have followed the example of my neighbor and taken a small piece of black electrical tape and covered up the section of her lab report that showed her cholesterol level. She could have pretended her risks didn't exist or she could begin to change her lifestyle and work with her physician to lower her risks.

Her lab report looked at a variety of health risks, and luckily for her, excessive body fat was not one of them. But, she still had some elevated health risks. Most of us are conditioned to think that if we have a healthy body weight, we are healthy. But that is simply not the case. Our beliefs about health risks are often not supported by reality. For example, the number one cause of death for smokers is not lung cancer, it's heart disease. If you smoke, the risk for heart disease goes way up. However, if you don't exercise regularly, your risk of heart disease is higher than if you were a smoker. Most of us have seen the health warnings and know that smoking is dangerous. But, the warnings about sedentary living are not as well known. We don't see them, hence we don't associate sedentary living with the same level of risk as smoking. Death and disease from sedentary living doesn't get the same level of attention as death and disease from tobacco use, so we naturally assume that smoking is worse for us.

The exact same association occurs with body fat. Individuals (68% of adults) who are overweight or obese can't hide the fact that they have elevated risks. The health risks of excessive body fat are tough to hide. The media has also done a good job of warning us about the risks associated with excess body fat so when we have excess body fat or see someone who does we are quick to think that their health is in jeopardy. On the other hand, when we see someone who has a healthy body weight we have no such thoughts about health risks. Indeed, we assume they are healthy, and we might even envy them. While it's true that health risks are low for those with a healthy body weight, there are a lot of other health risks that could actually put them at greater risk than those who are overweight. Don't be fooled into thinking that good health is determined just by body weight. It's not. Good health is determined by a variety of health risks, one of which is excessive body fat. If you are not overweight or obese congratulations—you've been able to avoid this one health risk. But, don't get too comfortable because there are many other health risks that you could easily have that may require some behavior change.

The New Normal

Lurking behind the obesity numbers shown in the graph is a cultural transformation that affects all of us, even those of us who are not struggling with excessive weight. The obesity epidemic is just one of the signs of this societal transformation. It's a sign we can all relate to because many of us (68%) struggle with excessive body weight. We experience it on a personal, intimate level. We see it all around us. We see others who are obese or overweight. We notice that children are heavier than they used to be. For those who travel abroad, one of the first things they notice when they return to the U.S. is that people here are really big.

Being overweight has become the new normal. Decades ago, it was normal to be thin. People did more physical labor and ate differently. Today, it seems that everyone has gained weight. As a people, we are bigger now than in any other time in human history. It is now abnormal to be thin, abnormal in the sense that most of us are not thin. Most of us are overweight and being overweight has become the new normal. This change in our perceptions and recognition of excessive weight has been found to be common. As we gain weight we slowly lose the ability to identify obesity, even when it is ourselves we are judging.[3] Parents are losing the ability to look at their children and determine if they are overweight or obese.[4] Increasingly, parents of overweight children underestimate their child's weight status or are not concerned about the risks associated with being overweight. The underestimations are even worse if the parents are obese. With fewer and fewer thin people around, we see mostly overweight adults and children. Because most of those we see are big, we get accustomed to people being large and large becomes normal. Years ago, obesity was the exception, and now it's the rule. Many times, the only ones standing out now are the ones who are lean and healthy. Do you remember the first time you saw someone talking on their cell phone while using one of those small ear pieces? It looked and sounded like they were carrying on a detailed conversation with themselves. You probably looked twice because you were sure they were talking to themselves. But, when you figured out what was going on, you likely laughed about it. If you saw someone doing the same thing today, you wouldn't think anything of it. It has become normal to see people having detailed conversations with themselves or at least with someone on their phone.

There is also a new normal in the way we eat. Over time, our relationship with food has changed. We don't eat the same way we used to. There are several aspects of food that have changed over the past few decades. These include our food quantity and our food quality. Quantity refers to increases in portion sizes; increases in the amount of food served at one meal, and the number of times we eat during the day.[5] Food quality really refers to what's in the foods we eat. Food close to its natural form is thought to have good quality, while highly processed food has low quality. Think about your great grandparents. What was the quality of their food? Most likely it included many foods that were locally grown, free from chemicals and close to their natural forms. Today, we have Coca-Cola, Hostess Twinkies and Spider-Man fruit snacks, which by the way don't contain any real fruit. Food quality also refers to the amount of energy or calories in the foods we eat. For example, a serving of cheesecake has a lot of calories, while a serving of vegetables has a lot fewer calories—it is less energy dense. Scientists refer to this as caloric or energy density. Foods that are high in fats have more calories per gram and have a higher energy density.

Decades ago, we consumed food in much smaller serving sizes. The food was also lower in caloric density and close to its natural form. Today, we drink milk, soda or juice instead of water. Grocery store shelves are lined with highly processed foods. Just take a look at the different types of breakfast cereals that can be purchased. Few of them even remotely resemble any food found in nature. These foods have become the new normal, they are the typical foods eaten by the average person. Just like healthy, thin people are sometimes seen as being abnormal, people who eat healthy foods can also be considered abnormal.

The shifts in our food choices have occurred slowly over many decades. The changes were so subtle that most often, we didn't even know that they occurred. This hasn't happened by chance; the shift to high density, poor quality foods has been deliberately planned and executed by the food industry. Brian Wansink is a food researcher who has spent his life testing how the food industry influences our eating habits and preferences. Here is a list of a few of the food and eating observations he has documented over the years:

- If you use a 10-inch dinner plate instead of a 12-inch dinner plate you eat 22% fewer calories.
- If you serve yourself, you will eat 92% of the food on the plate. If someone else serves you, you will eat much less.
- Low-fat labels lead people to eat 16-23% more total calories.
- Because of visual illusions, people pour 28% more into short wide glasses than tall ones.
- Greater variety in the assortment and colors of candy can double how much candy a person eats in one day.
- Labeling a food as being a Succulent Italian Seafood Filet can lead diners to much more favorably rate the taste than when it was simply labeled Seafood Filet.
- Elegance of dishes and the garnishes on plates increases a person's taste ratings of food.
- When foods are presented in a large bag or container people will eat more of it. (Think of a big bag of M&M's vs. tiny bags of M&M's)

An interesting aspect of Dr. Wansink's research is that after the studies were done, all the subjects denied that their eating behavior had changed. The change in the way foods are presented or served was so subtle they didn't even realize that their eating patterns had changed. When I see how the food industry has been carefully manipulating my eating and purchasing choices I kind of feel like I've been duped, falling victim to sneaky tricks they use to get me to eat more of their foods. All the while I don't even know they are doing it. It's like they got me to do something I didn't really want to do, (like eat an additional 570 calories per day) and I had no idea I was even being manipulated—sort of like being a parent of a 3-year-old.

Our food portions have also increased and most of us didn't realize these changes either. Rather than serve your meal on a plate, more restaurants now use platters. Plates are not large enough to hold all the food that is being served! Kid's meals often have more calories than a typical adult meal would have contained 30 years ago. It doesn't take a rocket scientist to figure out that people who are served more food, eat more food. Common sense would suggest this is true. Yet, scientists have done studies looking at this very issue and sure enough they have demonstrated repeatedly that when restaurants increase portion size, patrons eat more.[6] What these studies fail to point out is that restaurant patrons also get better value for their dining dollar. All those enormous servings mean that you get more food for the dollar. Smart consumers will split a meal with someone or only eat half and save the other half for later. The patrons who insist on consuming everything they are served are the ones who eventually end up on the graph shown at the beginning of this chapter. They become the overweight and obese—the new normal.

If it's true that we are all eating foods that are more energy dense—foods that have lots of calories—we should see evidence for this. Unless you've been carefully tracking everything you've been eating for your entire life, chances are you have no idea that your diet has changed and that you now eat a lot more foods that are energy dense. Cheese, cooking oils and high-fructose corn syrup are high density foods. The chart shown here shows the consumption of cheese, corn syrup and added fats for the past 50 or so years. The numbers on the chart are actually pounds per person per year. This data shows that the amount of cheese and added oils we eat has increased up to 200% and the amount of corn syrup we eat has increased 850%. In fact, the amount of corn syrup consumed in 2000 was about 85 pound per person per year.

I know what you are thinking. "I didn't eat 85 pounds of corn syrup in one year—that must have been someone else." I hear you and while it's true that these are averages and not all of it was eaten, the data is pretty accurate. So, if you didn't eat 85 pounds of corn syrup, and I'm pretty sure I didn't eat that much (at least I don't think I did). Then who did?

Per Person Consumption Of Cheese, Corn Syrup And Added Fats In The U.S. (pounds)

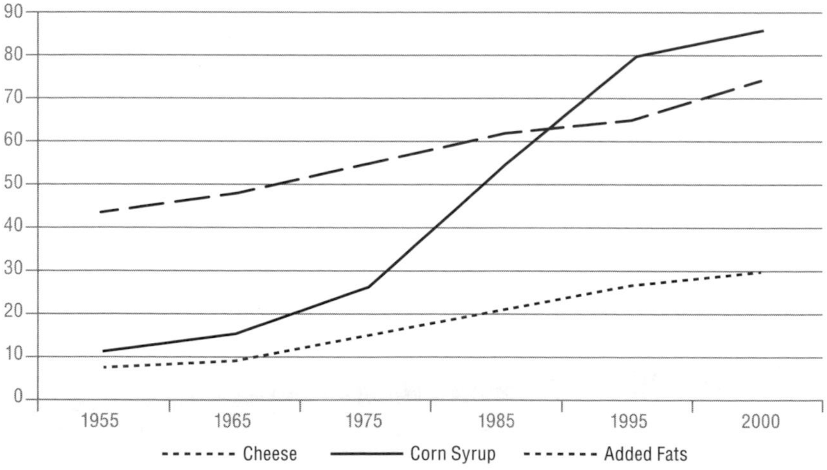

http://www.usda.gov/factbook/chapter2.pdf

Go to your kitchen and pull out a box or package of processed food. Something like a box of cereal, peanut butter, spaghetti sauce, yogurt or juice and look at the list of ingredients. There, you will likely find high-fructose corn syrup or corn sugar listed. These are corn-based sugars. Their production is subsidized by your federal tax dollars—they are 40% cheaper than white sugar and they are added to just about everything. Considering the fact that high-fructose corn syrup is hidden in many of the foods we eat, maybe you and I do eat 85 pounds per year. One of the best places to find high-fructose corn syrup is in soft drinks. If we as a nation are eating more high density foods, we should see increases in the amount of soft drinks being consumed. Fifty years ago the average person was drinking 10 gallons of soda a year (this information is not shown in the graph). Today, the average person consumes almost 50 gallons per year. Soft drink consumption has increased almost 500%. That's a lot of high-fructose corn syrup and a lot of extra calories. I like soda, I think it is delicious, but I try not to drink too much of it. However, I know a lot of people who drink a lot of soda and with most of that soda comes extra calories, extra pounds of fat, elevated health risks and the notoriety of being part of the fattest population in world history. It's hard to believe, but we now consume at least 50 gallons of soft drinks per person per year.

Of course, not all the foods we consume are getting eaten in greater quantities. In the past 50 years, fruit and vegetable consumption has remained relatively flat. These healthy, low energy density foods are still part of our American diet, but they are just maintaining their regular food status, while foods with high energy density become even more popular. There is one small ray of hope in the past 50 years of food consumption data. Consumption of whole grains has increased from 150 pounds to 200 pounds per year. Despite our increased desire for high-calorie foods, we seem to be eating more whole grains and that's a good thing.

Over the past 30 years, Americans have added an additional 570 calories to their daily diet.[5] The increase in calories has ultimately occurred because of two primary reasons. One, we eat more food, and two, the food we eat has more calories. These reasons describe the change that has happened in the amount of calories we consume, but it doesn't say anything about the calories we expend.

Everyone (who is living) expends calories just to maintain life. Our cells and organs use calories to work. The rest of the calories we expend are used to move our body. Physical activity is the main way we expend calories. Obesity trends are increasing, consumption of high calorie foods is increasing, but the number of people getting regular physical activity has not increased very much. It has only increased a few percentage points in the past decade. Even though we see more people out walking, riding bikes or visiting the gym, the number of people getting regular physical activity has increased very little. Maintenance of our body weight is pretty much defined by the number of calories we consume and the number of calories we expend. If physical activity trends are flat, the number of calories expended in physical activity hasn't changed much either. Add to this the increase in calories we all consume and the net difference has produced our current epidemic of obesity.

Why Should We Care?

I've been fortunate enough to work with companies and organizations all over the U.S. Recently, I spent time working for a large mining and marine company in the southern half of the U.S. They asked me to help them improve the health of their employees. I was curious as to why they were interested in helping their employees and their spouses have healthier lives. I ask this same question to every company I work with. Usually, I get the standard reply, "We need help reducing our health care costs," or "Our employees are not productive when they are struggling with health problems." But this time I got a different answer. The reason they wanted to start an employee wellness program was because their employees were dying.

The average U.S. adult lives to the age of 78. Many of these employees were dying before 65. They told me of at least eight cases where employees had passed away of sudden cardiac arrest, diabetes, cancer or strokes—all of them before the age of 65. This company has very expensive boats and equipment that require constant maintenance and upkeep. But the most expensive and important assets they have are their people. Decades of valuable work experience and knowledge are lost when employees die. Retirement accounts go untapped, grand children never get visited and families are left to make sense of the early loss. The early loss of key employees threatened the very viability of this company.

The first time an employee died, the company was in a sudden state of shock. Certainly, people can pass away unexpectedly. This is understandable; it's a normal part of life. But then it happened again. This time it was in another division of the company, but the outcome was the same. The devastating loss of valuable friends and coworkers left a gaping hole in the organization. It didn't just happen a few times, it kept happening. This company treats its employees very well. Few of them ever leave the company, so with very few people leaving, the average age of the employees is slowly climbing. With increasingly older employees working in an unhealthy part of the country the trend of premature death is likely to continue.

This company is located in the Deep South. Many foods are deep fried. Gravy is considered a beverage and over 60% of all employees smoke. Lifespans in this part of the country are not the same as the rest of the U.S. In parts of the south, lifespan is four to seven years shorter on average, and among these employees, lifespan is even shorter.[7] The main reason lifespan is shorter is because many of these employees have unhealthy behaviors. They may not eat healthy foods, may not exercise much and are likely to smoke. These behaviors cause blood pressure, glucose and cholesterol levels to elevate. They eventually develop life-ending chronic diseases like heart disease, cancer and diabetes and often they die 10 to 20 years before their time.

All this discussion about increases in our body weight, changes in our food quality and quantity, failure to improve exercise rates and having unhealthy behaviors doesn't mean much unless you are able to see where it all leads. This mining company in the south is seeing firsthand where it's going—to premature death for many of its employees. Clearly, it's worse in the southern half of the United States, but it's not confined to the south.

Here are a couple more charts to help you understand the seriousness of our unhealthy behaviors. The following map of the U.S. shows 2010 obesity rates on a state-by-state basis. Locate your state and you'll see that at least 20% of all adults are obese. The darkest states have obesity rates greater than 30%. Notice that with the exception of Michigan, the states with the highest rates of obesity are located in a swath that stretches from Texas to West Virginia. Don't be fooled into thinking that because your state isn't one of the darkest states you don't need to worry. Just wait a few years. In just a few short years, all the other states will catch up to the southern states.

Percent of Adults Who Are Obese (CDC)

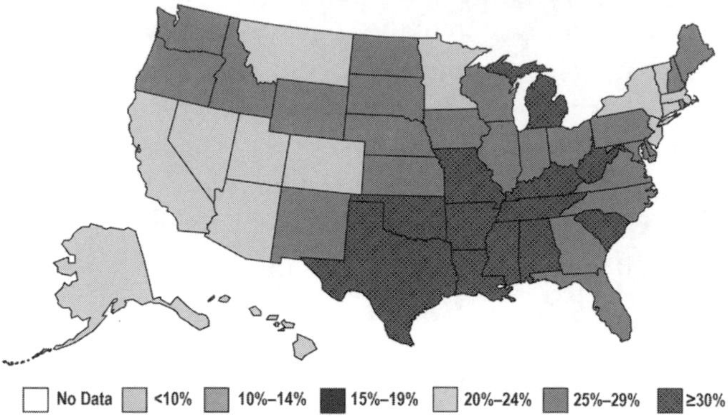

The second U.S. map shows the life expectancy for every county.[8] The residents of the darkest counties have a life expectancy from 62 to 71 years. The people in the lightest counties live much longer on average (75-80 years). There is almost a 20-year difference in life span between the different counties.

Live Span by County[9]

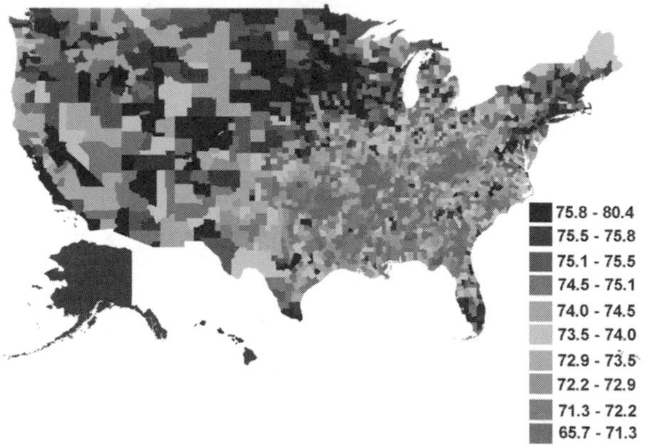

Compare these two maps. States with high obesity also have the shortest life expectancy. One quarter of all U.S. counties saw an actual reduction in life expectancy for women between 1997 and 2007, meaning that girls born today are expected to live shorter lives than their mothers. The men fared just as badly. Just like the obesity maps, the lowest life spans can be seen in counties that create a swath from Texas to West Virginia. The two maps are almost identical. To be fair, life span can be influenced by our gender, exposure to violence, infections like HIV, tobacco use and other factors, but the similarity between these two maps is striking.

In 1900, the average adult in the U.S. lived to about 45 years of age. Today, the average age at death is about 78 years. For the past century, life span in the U.S. has increased every year...until now. A reduction in life span of this magnitude is extremely rare in the developed world unless there is a catastrophic plague or war that results in widespread deaths. We haven't had any plagues and our wars have not been on American soil, and yet for the first time in the past century we're seeing reductions in life span in counties with the least healthy lifestyles.

The surveys used to create each map measured two completely different things: obesity and life span, and yet they look almost identical. That's because obesity and life span are both directly influenced by a third variable not shown on the maps: unhealthy behaviors. I could also share with you state-by-state maps showing the prevalence of smoking, poor diets or lack of exercise, but it would be a waste of paper because they all look just like the two maps on the previous page. It's worse in the Deep South, but within just a few years all areas of the U.S. will have the level of risk the south has now. The research is quite clear. Our unhealthy behaviors lead to elevated health risks, like obesity and high cholesterol. Elevated health risks lead to chronic diseases, which ultimately lead to a shortened life span.

Premature death as serious as it is, is just one outcome of our unhealthy lifestyles. There are many, many more reasons why you should be concerned about our future. Scientists who look at current trends and make predictions about the future have published some pretty frightening conclusions. Here's one in particular that really scares me.

There is an explosion of the number of people in the U.S. who have diabetes. The trend for diabetes prevalence looks a lot like the obesity trend at the beginning of this chapter. That's because obesity is the biggest single predictor of diabetes. Using the current and future trends in childhood obesity, researchers asked a single question: "What percentage of children born in the year 2000 will be diabetic before the age of 50?"[10] Among white children, 35% will be diabetic before the age of 50. The rate for black children is 43% and among Hispanic children, almost half (49%) will have diabetes before age 50. These predictions suggest that one-third to one-half of all children born in the year 2000 will have diabetes. If adults are already dying 10-20 years prematurely in the south, what will happen when all these diabetic children grow up? The same researchers demonstrated that anyone who is diagnosed with diabetes before age 40 will likely die 12 to 14 years early. So, if these predictions hold true, we are likely to see an even steeper decline in life expectancy.

But wait, something is not right here. A government report recently showed that life expectancy had reached an all-time high of 78.3 years.[11] The report provided clear proof that Americans are living longer now than at any other time. So, how could two different government reports show seemingly opposite conclusions? Both reports are correct. In the south, life span is getting shorter for many Americans, especially among minority women, but in other parts of the country—counties that are light colored, life span is getting longer. When the different counties are averaged together, the average for the nation shows an increase in life span. It appears that there are two sides to this story. First, our health behaviors have gotten worse over time; we've gained a lot of weight and different parts of the country are worse than others. Second, despite the unhealthy behaviors we all have, our life span keeps increasing. Believe it or not, there is an answer to this mystery.

Most of us are living longer, but we're doing so with chronic disease. We have chronic diseases, but because of medications and procedures like stenting, we've been able to keep the disease at bay for a few more years before we die.[12] The number of cases of cardiovascular disease, cancers and diabetes have not dropped. If anything, they've stayed the same or increased over time, which means we live longer, but we live with chronic disease. And though many have been able to delay death, they are living a long life with a chronic disease, which is a very unpleasant experience. The length of our lives may be increasing for some Americans, but because of chronic diseases (caused by a poor lifestyle) the quality of our lives is declining. Because of the lifestyles we live, the extra years we are seeing are often marred by loss of mobility and the ability to function physically.

Besides a poor quality of life, there is something more that comes with a long, not so healthy life—an enormous health care bill. I spend my days trying to help people adopt and maintain healthy behaviors. I like to say I've devoted my life to helping people use good nutrition, exercise and healthy living to prevent and avoid chronic diseases. That being said, I'm attuned to anything health-related that I come across or hear.

One evening I was driving home from work while listening to National Public Radio. During a break the announcer was listing all the companies that had provided financial support for their programming. The announcer caught my attention when he mentioned one sponsor in particular. Novo Nordisk is a $60 billion company with over 30,000 employees worldwide. It's a massive organization with a clear mission statement: "Diabetes treatment is our passion." Not diabetes prevention or eradication, diabetes treatment. Now, I'm sure they provide great products for the treatment of diabetes, but they are in business to make money on treating a disease that is 91% preventable. I don't blame them for anything. But like hospitals, doctors, pharmaceutical companies, insurance companies, malpractice lawyers and medical equipment manufacturers, their business model is entirely dependent on people getting chronic diseases. You and I see chronic diseases as difficult trials to be survived, and others see them as outstanding business opportunities. These opportunities add up to $2.5 trillion every year and of that amount, 70% is believed to be spent on the treatment of preventable chronic diseases.[13] Unhealthy behaviors lead to chronic diseases and the most expensive health care system in the world. Currently, the cost of health care in the U.S. is $14,000 per person per year and most of this is spent treating diseases that were caused by unhealthy lifestyles.

So, in addition to a shortened life span or a long life span with a poor quality of life, there is an enormous financial burden that is the direct result of our poor behaviors and subsequent chronic diseases. You and I pay the cost. Next time you buy a car know that a large part of the purchase price is to cover the health care cost of some worker and his family.

Enough Doom And Gloom

Okay, all this talk about getting fatter, dying early and having a long, poor quality life is pretty depressing. The goal of this book is not to drag you through these gloomy health trends only to leave you with a sense of hopelessness or despair. Yes, our health is bad and it's getting worse, but a growing ray of hope is breaking forth from within the shadows of the dismal data. This ray of hope is so strong and has so much potential that I quit my cushy job to help it gain strength.

I spent 20 years of my life working in universities as a professor. I had become a full professor and had earned tenure. Basically, if you have tenure you can't be laid off. It is the ultimate in job security. Combined with a good salary I could ride out the rest of my days in security and ease, teaching a few classes, writing a few papers and golfing in the afternoons. What a life! However, after 20 years behind the walls of academia, I decided to quit my job. I decided to walk away from the comforts, security and ease enjoyed by so many. I told my wife I was ready to be more involved in improving the health of all Americans. Rightly so, she and several of my colleagues were convinced I was nuts. Nobody leaves such a cushy job. Maybe I had lost my marbles. If what I have already described about the worsening state of our health is true, the future looks pretty bleak for millions of Americans.

I quit anyway, and I'll show you why. When consulting with people across the U.S., I meet people who, despite the pressures to be unhealthy, have managed to rise above the unhealthy environment to maintain a healthy diet, not smoke and participate in regular exercise. These people undergo a health transformation that will both extend life span and help them enjoy a long, high quality future. I call these people Island Natives.

Island Natives are people who have created and live on islands of health in order to avoid all the doom and gloom. I'm not referring to actual islands with tropical sands and turquoise seas. The islands I am referring to are more like safe havens: homes, businesses or communities, that despite being completely surrounded by a culture that promotes unhealthy behaviors, do everything necessary to make it easier to live a healthy lifestyle. The individuals (natives) who live on these islands still live in the real world. They have to balance work, family and the challenges of life just like everyone else. They live in the same neighborhoods and work at the same places we do, yet they are different. They have succeeded in being healthy while most of us fail. Throughout this book, I will share their strategies, challenges and victories. I do so because they show us an alternate way to live our lives, and there is much we can learn from them.

As gratifying as these stories are, they are just that: personal accounts of struggles to be healthy. I love to hear them, but I would have never quit my job just because I heard personal reports and inspirational before and after stories. I'm the most skeptical person I know. I want to see real data, studies that prove that people can really change behaviors, that health risks improve when they do, that chronic diseases are avoided and that life is really extended. The real reason I left academia is because the scientific evidence proves that healthy lifestyle change is effective. I quit so I could more effectively take this information to the masses where it can impact all Americans, not just the ones sitting in my classes.

We know enough now to improve public health more than in any other time in history. Cancer, heart disease, stroke, diabetes, erectile dysfunction, Alzheimer's disease, Parkinson's disease, liver disease and many, many other life-altering diseases are mostly preventable conditions. They don't have to happen. Life can be extended and quality of life can be dramatically improved. The research I've been conducting provides an obvious solution to so much suffering. I could keep my cushy job and hope people would read the studies and decide to change behaviors or I could leave and become part of a movement that can improve the health of all Americans— a mission, if you will, to transform public health. Enough research and studies have been completed. It's time to distribute the lifestyle change knowledge and tools that have been discovered to those who want to create a healthier, more enjoyable future.

Like my neighbor and his car, Americans are seeing a lot of white smoke; symptoms and signs of chronic disease, diabetes and obesity that all signal that something isn't right. The smoke isn't the problem; the real problem is something much deeper and more menacing. The first step to transforming our health is to solve this mystery. We will solve it and as soon as we do, the solution will become more obvious. Here's a hint…it involves islands of health.

Body Mass Index Table

	Normal						Overweight					Obese										Extreme Obesity														
BMI	19	20	21	22	23	24	25	26	27	28	29	30	31	32	33	34	35	36	37	38	39	40	41	42	43	44	45	46	47	48	49	50	51	52	53	54
Height (inches)	Body Weight (pounds)																																			
58	91	96	100	105	110	115	119	124	129	134	138	143	148	153	158	162	167	172	177	181	186	191	196	201	205	210	215	220	224	229	234	239	244	248	253	258
59	94	99	104	109	114	119	124	128	133	138	143	148	153	158	163	168	173	178	183	188	193	198	203	208	212	217	222	227	232	237	242	247	252	257	262	267
60	97	102	107	112	118	123	128	133	138	143	148	153	158	163	168	174	179	184	189	194	199	204	209	215	220	225	230	235	240	245	250	255	261	266	271	276
61	100	106	111	116	122	127	132	137	143	148	153	158	164	169	174	180	185	190	195	201	206	211	217	222	227	232	238	243	248	254	259	264	269	275	280	285
62	104	109	115	120	126	131	136	142	147	153	158	164	169	175	180	186	191	196	202	207	213	218	224	229	235	240	246	251	256	262	267	273	278	284	289	295
63	107	113	118	124	130	135	141	146	152	158	163	169	175	180	186	191	197	203	208	214	220	225	231	237	242	248	254	259	265	270	278	282	287	293	299	304
64	110	116	122	128	134	140	145	151	157	163	169	174	180	186	192	197	204	209	215	221	227	232	238	244	250	256	262	267	273	279	285	291	296	302	308	314
65	114	120	126	132	138	144	150	156	162	168	174	180	186	192	198	204	210	216	222	228	234	240	246	252	258	264	270	276	282	288	294	300	306	312	318	324
66	118	124	130	136	142	148	155	161	167	173	179	186	192	198	204	210	216	223	229	235	241	247	253	260	266	272	278	284	291	297	303	309	315	322	328	334
67	121	127	134	140	146	153	159	166	172	178	185	191	198	204	211	217	223	230	236	242	249	255	261	268	274	280	287	293	299	306	312	319	325	331	338	344
68	125	131	138	144	151	158	164	171	177	184	190	197	203	210	216	223	230	236	243	249	256	262	269	276	282	289	295	302	308	315	322	328	335	341	348	354
69	128	135	142	149	155	162	169	176	182	189	196	203	209	216	223	230	236	243	250	257	263	270	277	284	291	297	304	311	318	324	331	338	345	351	358	365
70	132	139	146	153	160	167	174	181	188	195	202	209	216	222	229	236	243	250	257	264	271	278	285	292	299	306	313	320	327	334	341	348	355	362	369	376
71	136	143	150	157	165	172	179	186	193	200	208	215	222	229	236	243	250	257	265	272	279	286	293	301	308	315	322	329	338	343	351	358	365	372	379	386
72	140	147	154	162	169	177	184	191	199	206	213	221	228	235	242	250	258	265	272	279	287	294	302	309	316	324	331	338	346	353	361	368	375	383	390	397
73	144	151	159	166	174	182	189	197	204	212	219	227	235	242	250	257	265	272	280	288	295	302	310	318	325	333	340	348	355	363	371	378	386	393	401	408
74	148	155	163	171	179	186	194	202	210	218	225	233	241	249	256	264	272	280	287	295	303	311	319	326	334	342	350	358	365	373	381	389	396	404	412	420
75	152	160	168	176	184	192	200	208	216	224	232	240	248	256	264	272	279	287	295	303	311	319	327	335	343	351	359	367	375	383	391	399	407	415	423	431
76	156	164	172	180	189	197	205	213	221	230	238	246	254	263	271	279	287	295	304	312	320	328	336	344	353	361	369	377	385	394	402	410	418	426	435	443

Source: Adapted from *Clinical Guidelines on the Identification, Evaluation, and Treatment of Overweight and Obesity in Adults: The Evidence Report*

CHAPTER 2

You Are A Caveman

TO SOLVE THE MYSTERY OF WHY SO MANY OF US HAVE SUCH POOR HEALTH, WE HAVE TO GO BACK IN TIME, WAY BACK. WE'LL START BY GOING BACK JUST ONE GENERATION, TO YOUR PARENTS. YOU INHERITED YOUR BODY FROM THEM. You likely share the same eye and hair color, you have a similar body shape and you may even share a similar voice and smile. Every aspect of your body was inherited from your parents. Even as a newborn infant you had features that mirrored your parents. These similarities don't stop at our features and skin, they go much deeper. You and your parents have the same stomach, brain, bones and blood. You are a genetic mix of your mom and dad; a physical replica of each, carefully blended together in such a way that every cell in your body can be traced to your parents. These similarities extend to your grandparents. Even though you are now two generations away from your grandparents, you still share the same physical traits and characteristics. Your eyebrows, teeth and pancreas are not really yours, they are actually the ones given to you by your parents, grandparents, great grandparents and so on. The further back we go the more we can see that our bodies really came from all those who preceded us.

If we are all just genetic replicas of our ancestors, then all of our cells, organs and tissues are not really ours—they were passed on to us by the generations of people who preceded us. How long have these body parts been moving from parent to child? When did it all start? Who were the first ancestors to start passing genetic code along to their children? The answers to these questions come with a lot of passion, depending on how the questions are answered. Strong feelings can be quickly aroused and many react swiftly to any information that runs contrary to long-held religious and cultural beliefs. I have no desire whatsoever to make this a discussion about religion or sacred scripture. My intent is to help you understand why our health is not as good as it should be and what we can do about it. To do so, I'm going to give you some things to think about. You don't have to agree or disagree; you just have to consider how the information may be impacting your health right now. So take a deep breath, exhale and let's have some fun with this.

Christians, Jews, Muslims and others have the creation story of Adam and Eve which describes the beginning point for our ancestors. I include myself with this group. I like the story of Adam and Eve. If it is taken literally we can use biblical genealogies to roughly estimate that they started having kids about 6,000 years ago. If it's true, then about 270 generations have passed to get from them to us. That means that our great, great, great, great (repeated 270 times) grandparents were Adam and Eve, and everyone on planet Earth has pretty much the same basic cells, organs and tissues that Adam and Eve had. This is one explanation of how it all started and one explanation about the origins of the physical body you and I possess. There is another answer to the "when did it all start?" question.

Newborn infants instinctively know that their mothers are equipped with breasts, nipples and a ready supply of life sustaining milk. All female mammals nurse their young. Just like women, men also have nipples and mammary glands (don't worry they are undeveloped and just don't work). Nipples in men, strange as they are, are just one quirky aspect of being human that suggest we really don't have a full understanding of our physical bodies and how we came into existence. In full disclosure, I really like the story of Adam and Eve, but I'm also a scientist and I really like the knowledge and information science can provide. I don't understand how everything fits together, but I'm comfortable with that. There are lots of things I don't fully comprehend. I don't understand how I can be traveling in my car at 65 miles per hour, talking on the phone to someone on the other side of the planet and have no delays or signal loss. When I think about it, it seems almost magical. Obviously there is an explanation, I just don't know what it is, nor do I understand it. Likewise, I can't explain how the story of Adam and Eve fits in with the discoveries made by science, but I'm okay with that. Someday we'll have it all figured out. I also do not know why men have nipples. But we do.

All of our bodies have remnants or evidence of a long and varied past that despite our lack of understanding, exist. These are called human vestiges, anatomical structures, traits or instincts that have lost most of their original function. Nipples on men are anatomical structures that no longer have any real function. We inherited them from our parents—every male has them, but they serve no real purpose.

The popularity of vampire movies has shown us another human vestige: fangs. We don't use the word fangs to describe human teeth; we have a kinder, less threatening word, canines. All of us have a set of upper and lower teeth that come to a point. These are our canine teeth. I have a wonderful yellow lab named Dixie. She has canines that look more like fangs. Hers are longer than mine, but the fact that we both have them is kind of weird. Fangs are really helpful when we are trying to bite something and not let it escape. Dixie does this when we play tug of war with a rag. A cat does this when catching a bird. I don't use mine much anymore because my meat comes already dead, fully cooked, layered between two pieces of bread and topped with fresh vegetables. I don't worry about my food escaping anymore. I still have my canine remnants though, just in case Dixie and I have to drag down some wild game.

The vertebrae in our spines start at the base of the skull and run the length of our backs ending with a little curly snippet at the end. It's called a tail bone. I have a tail bone. You have a tail bone. Dixie has a tail bone. She uses hers to communicate a wide range of emotions, feelings and temperaments. It doesn't matter if you are a human, another dog, or a cat; she always uses the international language of wag. Her tail never stops wagging. Sometimes I worry she is going to break it because she beats it so hard against things. I have similar emotions, I have the similar need to communicate with others, but unlike Dixie, my tail bone has lost its function. But I still have a little one.

Everyone has toe nails. Other than painting them, what do we use toe nails for? What purpose do they serve? We have finger nails too, they help us pick things up and scratch. We can scratch an itch or scratch an enemy. Scratch hard enough and you can draw blood. Dixie has finger nails and toe nails too, but hers are longer, thicker and curved. Hers are really claws, not just nails and she uses them to climb and dig. Tigers use them to hold and kill fleeing prey. Just like all other mammals, we have claws too, but we've pretty much lost our ability to use them for anything more than texting, removing slivers and looking pretty.

Right where your small intestine joins up with your large intestine is a little pouch-like structure called the appendix. Everyone has one. Most of the time we live our lives with little knowledge of or concern for our appendix until it becomes infected or inflamed. An inflamed appendix can be life threatening. Surgeons routinely remove the appendix once it becomes inflamed. You can live just fine with or without it and doctors and scientists have no idea why we even have one, yet we all do. Doctors prefer to leave it in if they can, not because it has some vital role, but because if you ever need some form of reconstructive surgery the appendix can be used to make tubes or pouches.

When Dixie sees other dogs or wild animals the hair on her back stands up. It makes her look bigger and meaner. Every hair follicle on her has a tiny muscle attached to it. When needed, she can make all these muscles contract at once and the hairs on her back stand straight up. When the muscles relax, her hair lays flat again. Have you ever had an experience that made the hair on the back of your neck stand up? If so, you are using your hair muscles, just like Dixie. The most common time we do this is when we get goose bumps. Goose bumps are nothing more than our hair follicles getting pulled upward by the same tiny hair muscles. We get goose bumps when we are cold, hoping to somehow get our hair to stand up and provide us with a better layer of insulation. Except there is one small problem. We no longer have much body hair. We still have the hair follicle and tiny muscles and we can still cause the muscle to contract when we are cold or scared, but unlike Dixie, we don't get much out of it because we no longer have much body hair. Everything but the hair is still there.

Nipples, canine teeth, tail bones, toe nails, an appendix and goose bumps are just a few of the remnants we possess. We have wisdom teeth, muscles we no longer use, membranes on our eyes and extra smell receptors. There are many examples of strange, anatomical structures in our bodies that we no longer use. We're like walking museums of ancient, but strange, anatomical and physiological remnants. Their very presence is hard to ignore. The fact that they exist in our bodies and in other mammals suggests that we may somehow all be connected, that through the passage of time we inherited these anatomical traits that are no longer needed in the world we now live in. It hints at the concept of evolution, but I don't want to use the "E" word. I'm going to leave that discussion for another time. I prefer to use the word "adapt" to describe how over time our bodies have changed to better cope with a changing environment and not everything in our bodies (vestiges) has been fully removed.

Very Old Brains, Too

Besides these physical vestiges to the past, we have also inherited some of our emotions, instincts and cognitive processing abilities from our ancient ancestors. One summer day I was working in my garden while Dixie wandered around my fruit orchard looking for dried fruit that had fallen to the ground. I watched her pick up several pieces of fruit and bury them in different locations around my property. As I watched her bury this dried fruit I started laughing because I knew there was no way she was ever going to dig them up and consume them at a later time. I know because in the past I've been digging in my garden and uncovered buried bones, chew toys and dried fruit that she had buried there before, but had neglected to recover or forgotten about. She's pretty good at burying food for later use, but not so good at digging it up again. The act of burying food for later consumption is called caching or hoarding. It was important in the ancient world where food was often scarce and it was important to keep the food hidden from other predators. Wolves and coyotes still do it, effectively, I might add. Dixie knows she is going to get fed twice a day, yet she continues to bury food. Most dogs continue to cache food even though the need to cache food ended a long time ago. Burying food for later use is an instinct, a basic behavior embedded deep in her genes and brain that she inherited from her parents even though survival no longer depends on it. I haven't seen any humans burying their food lately, but I have seen similar abilities or instincts in humans that suggest that we really do have ancient bodies living in a modern world.

Think of the last time you heard a talk or speech. What do you remember about what was said? If you have a really good memory you will likely remember a few disconnected ideas or thoughts. But if the speaker told a story, I'm confident that you would recall all of it, even the details. Humans have an incredible ability to recall stories. Most of us don't remember dates, names or to-do lists, but all of us remember stories. Researchers have suggested that this ability to mentally process, store and recall stories is a gift we all received from our ancient ancestors who didn't have sticky notes, flash drives or cameras. They used stories to remember extensive genealogies and family lineages. Verbal story telling was about the only way information was passed on from one generation to the next. Written language came much later in the history of humans, and even then, only the extremely privileged could read or write. For thousands of years stories were the only way to communicate large amounts of information from one person to another.

Somehow our brains adapted to this form of communication because we have a powerful, instinctive ability to remember them and repeat them to others. I speak to groups all over the U.S. and sometimes I get to speak to the same group again after a few years. Invariably, they don't usually remember what I spoke about last time unless I shared a personal story. For the audience, the story lives on as they can repeat it almost verbatim, but all the other words that came out of my mouth were processed, understood, and placed in short-term memory only to be automatically deleted after a while. Some have suggested that our reaction to music is another example of traits and characteristics we inherited from our ancient ancestors. The beating of drums causes a reaction in all of us, perhaps because we've been hearing drums and music for millennia. Some even believe that our facial emotions can be traced back to our ancient experiences.

We're All The Same

Now let's re-ask the earlier question, "How long ago did our earliest ancestors inhabit the earth?" The bible suggests it started about 6,000 years ago. That's one answer. But the presence of our strange anatomical remnants combined with tens of thousands of scientific studies suggest that perhaps our first ancestors were older than 6,000 years, much older. Drawings on cave walls, construction and even genetic testing on the remains of ancient humans suggest that our earliest ancestors could have been on the earth 2.5 million years ago.[1] Others suggest that humans started to appear in different places around the world 100,000 years ago. For our purposes, it doesn't matter which scenario you believe because the most important part to remember is that our ancestors lived a long time ago. We have the same bodies now, except our ancient bodies are out of place in the modern world in which we now live.

Just for the sake of argument we'll continue this discussion with the information science has provided. Lets' just say that our ancient ancestors started the human race 100,000 years ago. That means that since the beginning of man, there have been about 4,500 generations and our earliest relative would be your great, great, (repeated 4,500 times) grandfather. His name was probably Thor. His mate's name was probably Thelma and together they lived in a cave with other close relatives.

When you think about life 100,000 years ago, you may picture some pretty ugly humans living in caves and wearing animal skins. We are tempted to think that they were not the most intelligent creatures, completely unfamiliar with civility and social order. However, the discovery of handmade tools, paintings, artworks, formal burials and elaborate jewelry would suggest otherwise. They may have lived in a very different culture and environment, but mentally, physically, emotionally and perhaps even spiritually, they were our equals. My dog Dixie and I are not equals. She may want to be treated as an equal and we definitely consider her to be family, but we are not equals. We share some of the same anatomy and even though we share most of the same DNA, we're just not the same. She is a dog, a very smart one at that, and I am a human. But I am equal to my ancient Paleolithic ancestors, equal in every way down to the tiniest organelle in the tiniest cells of my body. Culturally, you and I are citizens of the 21st century, but genetically we are cavemen. I know this may be a hard concept to grasp because your mind is telling you that you're different, but your body still thinks it's a caveman. We'd like to think we are a sophisticated, highly intelligent, modern being, but the physical remnants of a much older time can still be seen in us in the various vestiges our bodies possess. These bodily remnants of a different time and place are reminders that our bodies are the products of an older, different era. The body you received from your parents isn't your parent's body, nor your grandparent's body. It is the body that was developed for you by thousands of generations of your ancient ancestors who lived very different lifestyles. Your pancreas, eyes, liver, muscles and brain are not yours; they are a legacy or a gift from those who came before you. They are the culmination of 100,000 years of adaptation to different foods, weather, traditions and environments.

Obviously all humans are not the same, there are subtle differences in race, skin color, facial features, height and hair color, but even with these small differences all humans are 99.5% genetically identical. There is very little genetic variation within the human race. Likewise, the human gene pool changed very little over the past 100,000 years.[2] Human genes have not changed much for 100,000 years and even though humans today live in very different environments and locations, the gene pool is still almost identical. Humans are mostly the same across the world and across the eons of their existence. Not just you and I, but every human on the earth today possesses a body that is similar to every other body on the planet including the bodies of our ancestors.

Believe it or not, all this information is important when trying to understand how we can have a healthy, long and high quality life. If you agree that your body is an inheritance from ancient times, it will force you to look more closely at the environment and society it developed from. During those 100,000 years of human adaptation, what did our ancestors eat? How much did they exercise and if our modern world has changed so much, won't our bodies just adapt to the new foods and lifestyles we throw at it?

What's For Lunch In 100,000 BC?

Let's look at this discussion with a slightly different perspective. Let's pretend that 100,000 years of human existence is equal to one 24-hour day. Under this analogy, the 100,000 year period would start at midnight and end 24 hours later at midnight. With this perspective the Ice Age which ended 10,000 years ago would have ended at about 9:30 in the evening—almost at the end of the of our 24-hour period. Christ would have been born at 11:12 p.m., just a few minutes before the end of the period. White sugar has only been part of our diet for about 200 years. White flour has only been publicly available for about 150 years and the most widely-consumed sweetener, high-fructose corn syrup, has only been around for about 45 years.[3–5] White sugar, white flour and high fructose corn-syrup are dietary newbies showing up in the last 12 minutes of the day. The Internet which many of us find to be an indispensable tool would have been around for the last 12 seconds! With this perspective we can see several important facts about diet and human history. Diet and physical activity patterns of our ancient ancestors have remained relatively unchanged for almost all of human history. Only in the most recent years have humans seen dramatic changes in the foods we eat, technology and all the enhancements that accompany the modern age. For most of the 100,000-year history of the human race our diets were pretty consistent and predictable. Even though all our ancient ancestors have been dead for thousands of years, we know what they ate.[6]

There are three ways to determine what people were eating tens of thousands of years ago. The first way is to look for people who still live that way. Researchers have carefully identified and studied hunter/gatherer populations from around the world. Aboriginal peoples have been documented on every continent and in various environments around the world. By combining all this research, we can create an accurate picture of what a typical ancient hunter/gatherer ate. A second way is to study the remains and living environments of Paleolithic peoples. Excavation sites are common throughout Europe, Africa and Asia. By carefully studying left over bones, tools and prehistoric trash piles some rough estimates of dietary practices can be provided. The last way is to actually analyze prehistoric bones. Using some sophisticated equipment, researchers can determine what percentage of an ancient person's diet came from animals and plants.[7]

When data from all three methods are combined an interesting snapshot of our ancient diet appears. It is estimated that about 50% (the range is 35 to 70%) of our ancient ancestors' diet came from animals. The other 50% came from plants.[8] That's right, our hunter/gatherer ancestors really were hunters first, and gatherers second. Most of the men were likely busy tracking and killing wild game, while the women gathered roots, berries, fruits and other plant foods. For many years, researchers and the public assumed early humans ate mostly plants, but the total amount of research points to a range of diets with the average being about a 50/50 split between animal and plant foods. Obviously, there are regional differences around the globe. For example, Inuit societies live on 99% animals because in extreme arctic climates there are no plants. Likewise, some foraging tribes eat predominately more plants. I'm guessing a few of you reading this book right now are hard core carnivores, and are excited to tell your friends and family that today is the best day of your life because you just read that your body was specifically designed to eat meat and that eating a lot of meat is the pathway to good health. Not so fast modern meat eaters of America! Your excitement is premature. The meat eaten by your ancient ancestors is not the same meat you and I eat today. There is a big difference.

Not Thor's Burger

In ancient times, all animals were raised in the wild. Meat that was eaten came from animals that consumed other animals and plants found in the same ecosystem. Today, most Americans eat three main meats: beef, poultry and pork. In the past 100 years, cattle free-ranged and would take four to five years to reach a slaughter weight of 1,200 pounds. Today, those same cattle are fed in a feedlot, injected with growth hormones and reach the same slaughter weight in just 14 months. Today, 99% of all beef is produced from grain-fed, feedlot cattle.[9] The rapid growth seen in cattle has been duplicated with chicken and pork. The combination of a high grain diet, little exercise and artificial growth hormones can produce a ready-to-slaughter animal in a fraction of the time with a more favorable taste. In these animals, excessive body fat is stored in muscle cells giving meat the tender, fatty flavor preferred by consumers. Though our ancient ancestors ate more meat than we do, it was a very different type of meat.

Free-ranged cattle and wild game have less saturated fat, higher amounts of good fats and no artificial hormones. The meat we now consume has much higher amounts of saturated fat because it is mixed with liquid smokes, nitrates, sodium, sugar and spices to make processed meats like sausage, bacon, bologna and hot dogs. No doubt about it, the meat consumed by most Americans is very different from what our ancestors consumed. The meat we eat is still animal protein, but it's not quite the same. Regular consumption of our meat is now linked to certain cancers and cardiovascular diseases.[10]

The same differences exist in the consumption of fish. Man has been consuming fish since the beginning of the human race, and back then it was wild, organic and a vital component of their diet. Fish consumed today is rarely wild caught and if it is, it may run the risk of chemical contamination. I have the privilege of living in the beautiful Rocky Mountains. My state has the reputation of being clean and environmentally friendly. Fresh fish can be found in just about any body of water and yet of the 199 lakes and reservoirs here, 19 have mercury levels so high that the state advises anglers not to consume the fish they catch there.[9] Though some sources of fish may not be healthy, overall, the benefits of consuming fish outweigh any risks of exposure to chemicals and they should be consumed as part of a healthy diet.[12]

Most of the processed foods and meats we eat today are so delicious because they are loaded with salt. Of the 9 grams of salt we consume each day on average 75% of it comes from salt added during the processing of food. The rest is salt we deliberately add or is salt that occurs naturally in the foods we eat. But it wasn't always this way. Salt simply was not used until around 6,000 BC when some clever Chinese and Spanish folk figured out how to mine and use salt to preserve meats. The best evidence to date shows that our early ancestors did not add salt to the foods they consumed simply because they did not have access to it. Today, we've become accustomed to salty foods and in many ways we crave salt.

Breads, grains, rice and starchy vegetables have become such a staple of the world's food supply today that we can hardly imagine a time when humans did not eat them. But cereal grains were rarely consumed by humans until the last 10,000 years. The time before cereal grains is called pre-agricultural because until then plants were not planted, grown or harvested in a systematic fashion. Everyone was truly hunting and gathering. Once they figured out how to plant and harvest, the work of gathering probably got a little better organized. For most of human history, grains were not available in abundance. Even when they did become available they were not the processed grains we consume today. In fact, we don't eat grains today; we just eat the refined carbohydrates in the center of the grains. With modern milling practices, what used to be a whole grain has been stripped of its fiber and husk leaving just the white carbohydrate flour. Over 85% of all the grain we eat today is in the form of highly refined flour—a stark difference from the earlier grains our ancestors consumed.

Are you familiar with Lucky Charms breakfast cereal? Lucky Charms cereal is made from oats, but you wouldn't know it unless you carefully examined the ingredients. General Mills, the manufacturer of Lucky Charms, calls them a whole grain, frosted oats cereal and boasts that they are "Magically Delicious."

Here are the exact ingredients of Lucky Charms:

Lucky Charms Ingredients

Oat flour, marshmallow bits (sugar, modified corn starch, corn syrup, dextrose, gelatin, calcium carbonate, yellow 5&6, blue I, red 40, artificial flavor), sugar, corn syrup, corn starch, salt, calcium carbonate, color added, trisodium phosphate, zinc and iron (mineral nutrients), vitamin C (sodium ascorbate), a B vitamin (niacinamide), artificial flavor, vitamin B6 (pyridoxine hydrochloride), vitamin B2 (riboflavin), vitamin B1 (thiamin mononitrate), vitamin A (palmitate), a B vitamin (folic acid), vitamin B12, vitamin D, wheat starch, vitamin E (mixed topopherols) added to preserve freshness.

Now, imagine you were a caveman and you came across a box of Lucky Charms. You'd have to be impressed with the colorful marshmallow bits. After you carefully examined the various parts of the cereal you'd give it a taste. Just one handful would be enough for 100,000 years of bland tribal foods to get rejected. The refined oat flower mixed with sugar, corn syrup and more sugar would produce a taste only the Gods could have created. No wonder kids ask for more. Lucky Charms is a good example of a food that has undergone a level of processing that could not be further from what our ancestors consumed. Even though a few oats that are in Lucky Charms are actually whole oats (the shell, germ and starch of the oat kernel) this cereal is far from being a whole food.

All the sugar and sweeteners in Lucky Charms are modern inventions. Sugar production was first seen in India around 500 BC, but it took until the late 1800s before sugar was available to the masses. Today, the average American consumes 66 pounds of refined sugar each year. But, there's more. We also eat an additional 85 pounds of corn sweeteners. Combined, we eat 151 pounds of sweeteners per person per year.[13] Put another way, in one year we consume over 260,000 calories from sweeteners—a food that until just 150 years ago did not exist. Before the arrival of sugar, the only concentrated sugar available to humans was honey. Compared to our ancient ancestors the addition of sweeteners to our food supply has dramatically altered both the quality and the quantity of calories we consume. As a result of this unprecedented change, we have placed pressures on our Paleolithic body that it was never designed to handle.

To be sure, the types of meat we now eat, the addition of excessive salt and refined flour, and an enormous of amount of sweeteners have created a modern diet that is increasingly foreign to our ancient bodies. Unfortunately, it gets worse. Like the advent of agriculture, the advent of dairy products into the human diet is also a relatively recent occurrence. For 100,000 years, our ancestors' children consumed their mother's milk until the age of two or three. Eventually, their mother's milk dried up and the children made the transition to whole foods. For most of human existence, the consumption of milk ended when suckling stopped. It is easy to forget that there were no domesticated animals for most humans. There were no cows or goats to milk, just a lot of wild animals who weren't very interested in being milked. We have transitioned away from a diet completely void of all dairy products to one today that includes 30 pounds of cheese, 3 pounds of cottage cheese, 28 pounds of ice cream, 23 gallons of milk and 32 pounds of various dairy ingredients per person per year.[13]

As you may recall from the chart in Chapter 1, we consume more cheese now than at any other time. We put cheese on everything. What makes dairy products so appealing to us is the taste. Compared to foods acquired from hunting and gathering, dairy products are rich and creamy in flavor and are loaded with calories and saturated fat. Dairy products are big business in westernized societies with powerful, well-funded lobbyists.

I'm not a member of the nutrition community that has labeled milk and dairy products as foods that should never be eaten. I believe that the available research on the benefits and risks of consuming dairy products has been unduly influenced by those who profit financially from the sale of dairy products. More on this later, but suffice it to say that consumption of low-fat dairy foods in moderation strikes a nice balance between enjoying the taste of dairy without significantly increasing the risks of disease.

However, dairy consumption by the average American is not moderate nor is it low fat. The typical American consumes enough high-fat dairy and cheese to make their Paleolithic bodies struggle to maintain ideal health. This struggle gets even worse when we add extra fats from refined oils and spreads.

We may not often think about how our food gets to our table, but if you were to process all of your food yourself it would quickly become obvious that the amount of effort to get cooking oil, shortening or margarine is enormous. Olive oil can be obtained by pressing the olives, but when was the last time you pressed rapeseed to get Canola oil? Most of us don't even know what rapeseed is, let alone how it is grown, harvested and used to make cooking oil. Refined vegetable oils are a product of the Industrial Revolution. Thor and Thelma (our ancestors) could only dream of fried catfish and hushpuppies. They simply didn't have the technology or ability to make oils. Of course we do have the technology and we can't seem to get enough of it. It's right up there with sugar and corn syrup with most of us eating about 75 pounds a year. We use it in baking and frying and there is a huge variation in the quantity consumed depending on where you live in the U.S. In the south everything is fried, in California French fries are about the only commonly consumed fried food and in the Paleolithic world nothing was fried. There are so many calories in oils that you can use them to make biodiesel to power automobiles and trucks. In China farmers are growing rapeseed to make both cooking oils and vehicle fuel. The transition from a diet void of extra oils to one flush with oils is accompanied by chronic disease.

The table shown here lists the various foods consumed today that were almost entirely unavailable to our ancient ancestors.

Typical Foods Unavailable To Our Ancient Ancestors

Dairy Products	Cereal Grains	Refined Sugars	Refined Vegetable Oils	Others
whole milk	whole grains	table sugar	cooking oils	alcohol
low-fat milk	refined grains	corn syrup	shortening	salt
cheese		glucose	margarine	
butter		syrups		

These foods did not exist at that time. You will recall that our ancient ancestors had a diet that was about 50% animal and 50% plant-based. Contrast that to today's diet where the typical American gets 65% of calories from sugars, fats and refined grains, while meat is at 13% and dairy products make up 9% of calories. Fruits and vegetables, beans and nuts make up the remaining 13%.[14]

Consumption of animal products in the ancient world has been replaced with foods made of fats, sugars and flour, while the plant portion of the ancient diet has been cut by 75%. These may not seem like big differences, but over a lifetime the differences in the quality and quantity of food we eat makes a very real difference, one that can shorten your life by decades.

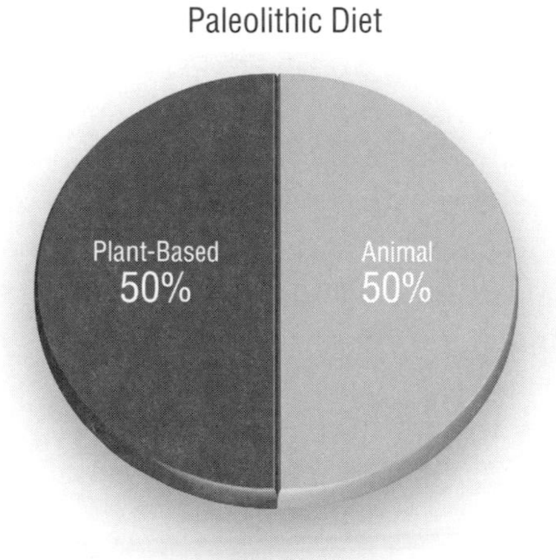

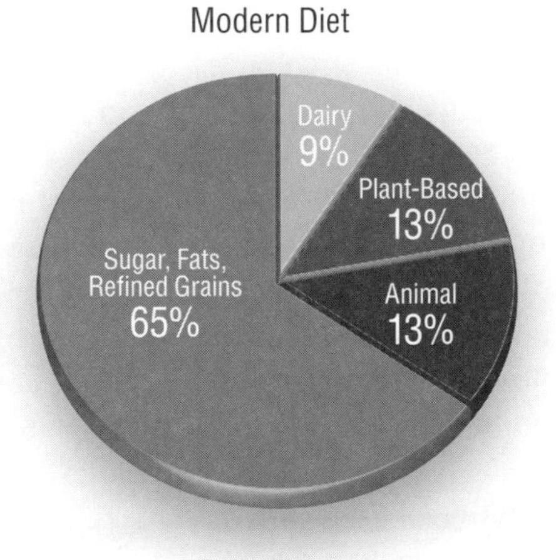

No Paleolithic Couch Potatoes

The dietary differences between ancient and modern humans are dramatic and these differences are believed to be responsible for many of the chronic diseases Americans experience today. Compared to our ancestors there are also differences in the amount of physical activity we get. Using many of the same methods to study ancient diets, paleontologists have estimated how much physical activity would be required for the typical hunter/gatherer.[15]

It doesn't take a Ph.D. to quickly realize that our caveman ancestors got a lot of physical activity. Take away all mechanical devices like cars, planes and bicycles and about the only thing left to help us find and gather food is our own two feet. Our ancestors didn't have the luxury of being sedentary because not moving meant not eating and eventually death. For them, life was about moving and only resting when they could. With the exception of the very young and the very old, sustained daily physical activity was a requirement for survival. For us it's about resting as much as possible and moving as little as possible, like when we have to get out of our chair because the television remote is on the other side of the room. Compared to us, our ancestors were extremely fit. They had a combination of both muscular strength and cardiovascular endurance because they had no mechanical or labor-saving devices to reduce the amount of energy needed to work. Today we may call this type of endurance, strength and flexibility training "cross training" but back then it was called "living".

A typical day may have included gathering plant food, building shelters, building tools, walking long distances over hills and fields to hunt, and carrying meat and logs. It is estimated that they covered a distance of 5 to 10 miles every day.[16] They could run when needed, dance for pleasure and tradition, dig for food, butcher meat and tend to the young. The women would gather foods, wood and water from long distances and often while carrying their young. By carefully studying aboriginal peoples today, some anthropologists estimate that ancient mothers physically carried their young until about the age of four years, covering a walking distance of almost 3,000 miles during this time period.[17]

With so much physical exertion required just to survive, our ancient ancestors developed stronger bones and muscles, and their hearts, lungs and circulatory systems became more efficient and faster at delivering oxygen and nutrients to the cells of their bodies. In essence, their bodies became accustomed to doing hard physical labor and covering long distances by walking and running. Fortunately, you and I have the same adaptations, but few of us actually provide our bodies with the level of physical activity it is built for.

Contrast ancient lifestyles to how we live today. Many of us are stressed out, sleep deprived, over fed, over stimulated and sedentary. Other than the need to eat, sleep, stay warm and reproduce, we have very little in common with our Paleolithic ancestors. Instead of gathering wood and tracking wild game, we have Facebook, Monday Night Football, (watching only, not playing) texting, driving and fast food restaurants with drive-thru windows where we can hunt down a precooked, slightly seasoned slab of meat wrapped in a toasted sesame seed bun. We get to bring home fresh kill without even having to exit the vehicle.

Not So Fast

It's important to try to realign our nutrition and physical activity behaviors with our ancient ancestors, but that's about as far as we need to go in trying to copy their ways of living. Our ancient ancestors lived extremely hard and short-lived lives. Estimates suggest that the average life span was only 35-40 years and many failed to survive childhood.[18] They almost never suffered from chronic diseases like we do because they had healthy lifestyles and rarely lived long enough to develop any chronic disease. They struggled just to provide for the basics of food, clothing and shelter. You and I will likely die of cardiovascular disease and cancer, while our ancestors died mainly from infectious diseases and accidents. Every day they labored to keep from being killed by predators or their enemies. To them, common daily accidents or a simple infection could be deadly because they had no access to the excellent medical care you and I take for granted today. Their lives were very, very hard. They struggled to survive and despite their ideal nutrition and active lifestyles they died young. We should appreciate all they did to help us have the lives we have today, but beyond their nutrition and exercise habits, there's not much to be envied.

If we could travel in a time machine that could take us back to the Paleolithic past we'd be able to actually experience what life would have been like in that ancient world. As amazing as this experience would be it wouldn't compare to doing it in reverse. If we could transport our ancient ancestors from their early human era to our modern day I'm pretty sure there would be some explaining to do. Rather than gather wood, start a fire and cook some food, all we have to do is place it in the microwave and push the button. While our ancestors had to regularly walk and hike to gather roots, berries and fruits, we spend our energy driving around the parking lot looking for the parking stall closest to the store we are trying to enter. Once parked, we do have to actually get out of our seats and walk. Carry containers of water from the stream? Not anymore. We just open the tap or better yet, get a drink from a disposable cup with 64 ounces of diet Coke and pick up some beef jerky at the checkout counter.

Our ancestors would gather logs to put on the fire while you and I would simply turn up the thermostat. Rather than physically dig for roots or tubers, we get our roots (potatoes) by digging for loose change to cover the cost of our 99 cent container of value French fries. Instead of carrying young children on our backs, we use a rear facing car seat with optional video display, four speaker surround sound and a collection of plastic kid's meal toys complete with plastic dinosaurs to remind us of an earlier period in Earth's history.

Despite our body's capacity to do hard, daily physical labor we subject it to a society where labor is shunned and the need for physical effort has been nearly eliminated. Genetically our hearts, lungs and vessels are ancient; they are used to being subjected to exercise and physical movement and when that doesn't happen, the processes that lead to chronic diseases begin.

New World-Old World Discord

Cardiovascular disease, stroke, diabetes and cancer are the result of the disconnect between the way we treat our bodies today and the way they were anciently designed to operate.[18] For example, today we eat highly processed, calorie-dense foods that are digested quickly. Unlike whole foods, highly processed foods are quickly digested and absorbed into the blood stream. This rapid absorption causes a spike in the amount of sugar and fats in our blood. This causes a condition called oxidative stress, which leads to inflammation in the artery walls. In response, the body deposits plaque and calcium in the artery walls eventually leading to stroke and heart disease.[19] This type of inflammation is a primary predictor of cardiovascular disease. Our ancestors did not get this inflammation because they did not eat this way. They consumed minimally processed high-fiber plants like vegetables, fruits, legumes and nuts. These foods take longer to digest, and introduce sugars, fat and nutrients into the blood stream over a longer period of time without causing inflammation. Cardiovascular disease is just one of the diseases that is directly related to our modern diet and lifestyle.

The modern development of diabetes is almost identical to the development of cardiovascular disease. Lack of physical activity and consumption of processed foods causes a spike in blood sugar. To clear the excess sugar from the blood stream the pancreas releases insulin. Insulin's job is to carry blood sugar from the blood into the cell. In response to a big spike in blood sugar, the pancreas releases a large dose of insulin causing a spike in insulin. Current research suggests that the constant need to produce large amounts of insulin wears the pancreas out, weakening its ability to produce insulin. At the same time, muscle cells, which are mostly sedentary, don't need much sugar. For some reason, cells begin to stop recognizing insulin when it comes knocking with more sugar. This is called insulin resistance, which means that our cells begin to resist insulin. Technically, the cell walls stop recognizing insulin and prevent it from entering to release its load of sugar. The ability to produce insulin is reduced while at the same time our cells stop recognizing it. The net result is elevated blood sugar and a diagnosis of insulin resistance or worse, diabetes. *Right now as you read these words, this exact process is happening to 35% of adults in the U.S. who are currently diabetic or who have insulin resistance.*[20] It is perhaps the most striking example of the discord between the nutrition and physical activity culture we have today and the ancient culture to which our bodies are adapted.

The processing of our food has another downside. Whole foods (fruits, vegetables and legumes) have specialized cancer and disease-fighting chemicals called phytochemicals. When we eat phytochemicals it's believed that they help protect our bodies from cancers, hardening of the arteries, strokes and even wrinkles. Anciently, our diets included large quantities of these health-promoting chemicals. Today, refined grains have mostly replaced much of the fruits, vegetables and whole grains we used to consume.

We Are Stuck

We could ignore this entire chapter if the human body were able to quickly adapt to its constantly changing environment. During the course of 100,000 years the human body has adapted to a consistent diet of animal products and plant foods and a daily need for constant physical activity. The process of change and adaptation takes tens, maybe even hundreds of thousands of years. Changes in our skin color, eye color and other physical features do occur. Just look around at the diversity within the human race and you can see evidence of these changes, but what you don't see is the time it takes for these changes to occur. In a very short amount of time human nutrition has undergone massive changes, an amount of time far too short for us to adapt to. If human physiology and anatomy could adapt more quickly, we would see dramatic changes in our abilities to digest new foods and perhaps less chronic disease.

Take alcohol consumption for example. There is evidence that alcohol was being prepared by humans as far back as 10,000 BC. For 10,000 years the human body has been exposed to the effects of alcohol, no doubt some more than others. And yet for 10,000 years our livers have failed to find improvements in alcohol digestion. It takes just as long now to break alcohol down as it did 10,000 years ago. We have been unable to adapt. Research shows no evidence of physiological adaptation in any part of our bodies over the past 10,000 years—even exposure to agriculture has not caused us to adapt.[18] In a sense, we are stuck in time, frozen in an ancient body while all around us the world is changing at a startling pace. Our challenge is to balance the opportunities of the new with limitations of the old. Right now many of us are failing this challenge, and based on our current trends it is bound to get worse. It's not easy, but it is doable, just like this Island Native shows us.

Island Native

My name is Conrad William. I'm 51 years old and work as a steel worker in Monroe, Louisiana. I always took pride in my health because I felt like it was the right thing to do. I didn't smoke and I was physically active at my work. With encouragement from my employer, I got a physical and had my blood screened. I was shocked to learn that I had high cholesterol, high blood pressure, was pre-diabetic and obese. I was overwhelmed by the news. I didn't want to take medications, but I realized that I had to change my lifestyle or shorten my life. My doctor told me I had to give up my Oreo habit. I was used to eating large portions, lots of fried foods and nine Oreos every day.

I learned that I could use alternatives to my unhealthy foods. For example, instead of white bread for sandwiches I could choose whole wheat and use 1% milk instead of whole milk. To help me stop eating the foods that weren't good for me I stopped bringing them home. "Out of sight, out of mind" became my new strategy for eating healthy. That's not always easy because here in Louisiana we love to eat fried food. I also knew that I needed to improve my physical activity habits. Once my company finishes a project we move to another one, so I travel a lot with my work. I travel with some weights and other packable exercise equipment that I can use no matter where I am. Even when working I try to stay active by working more vigorously for longer periods of time.

My motivation is my personal desire to be healthy. Most of the time I'm doing this alone, but my girlfriend supports me. She will run with me and when we're together we cook healthy meals. She too has decided to be healthy and together we support each other. Once I decided to change, I never looked back. I take no medications, and just by changing my life, I'm no longer pre-diabetic and I no longer have high blood pressure. In fact, I can now outrun the younger guys I work with. If I could say one thing to people who want to change I would say, "Be true to yourself." By that I mean if you truly want to live longer, you need to change. If you really want it, it's yours for the taking.

CHAPTER 3

The Real Problem

EVERYONE KNOWS SOMEONE LIKE MY FRIEND PAUL. HE'S MARRIED, BUSY WITH HIS CAREER, HAS SOME CHILDREN AND AN EXTRA 50 POUNDS OF BODY FAT TO CONTEND WITH. I've watched him lose a bunch of weight only to see it all gradually come back. He used a healthier diet of whole foods, in smaller portions and regular exercise to get the weight off. Within 12 months of losing the weight he slowly migrated back to his old eating and exercise habits and naturally the weight came back. Paul is not alone in his struggles to lose weight and maintain weight loss. Researchers have carefully followed participants of 17 different weight loss studies. After three years, 85% of those who lost weight regained almost all of it back.[1] Like Paul, they were successful initially, but after the weight loss program ended their resolve weakened and their battle to maintain a healthy weight was eventually lost. Of course, even though most people (85%) fail, 15% of people do succeed. These successful 15% have similar career and family obligations, they live in the same neighborhoods and environments and even though they feel the exact same pressures to go back to their old ways, for some reason they don't. Unlike the unsuccessful majority, they are somehow able to withstand the influences that impacted them in the past.

How can it be that despite the variety of weight loss programs, books and interventions available so few people are able to lose weight and maintain that loss? So many weight loss programs claim to have the solution, yet so many people fail to reach and maintain a healthy weight. Despite the efforts of the $61 billion a year weight loss industry, Americans have more body fat now than any other time in human history. How can we be spending so much time, money and energy trying to have healthy lifestyles only to see our weight and health status slowly get worse? Our failure to successfully control body weight is just one example of how complicated it is to have a healthy lifestyle.

The Mystery

This truly is a mystery. I've already demonstrated that our ancient bodies were never intended to be used in our new food and exercise free environment, but our Paleolithic bodies are only part of the poor health equation. To figure out this mystery, let's do a little experiment. I want you to think about what you ate for your last meal. It could be breakfast, lunch or dinner—it doesn't really matter. Take a second and make a mental list of all the different foods you consumed. See if you can also remember how much you ate. Got it? Now ask yourself this question. Why did you eat those foods in those quantities? For example, I'm thinking of the Malt-O-Meal, whole wheat toast and banana I had for breakfast. Why Malt-O-Meal? Why not eat a bowl of oatmeal, or biscuits and gravy? The decision process we use to decide what to eat at a meal is way more complex than you ever imagined. Taste, cost and convenience are the most common factors people list, but in addition to these, there are several other factors involved in your decision-making process. Your choice of which food to eat is swayed by your ability to cook, knowledge of how to shop for bargains, your age, gender, marital and financial status, where you live and the season of the year. If you eat lunch at school or work, the choice of which foods to prepare was made by someone else. You had no control over which foods were available, only which foods you ultimately selected. Family traditions have a huge impact on food decisions. My decision to eat Malt-O-Meal was no doubt influenced by the taste, but also by all the Malt-O-Meal commercials and advertisements produced by the manufacturer. Most of these advertisements were popular when I was a small child. I don't remember any of them, but I'm confident that my mother purchased Malt-O-Meal after seeing a few commercials. She brought it home one day, and the taste keeps coming back to me 50 years later. The aggressive marketing of the food industry has an enormous influence on what we eat. Even the government has a tremendous influence on what we eat every day. For example, the U.S. government subsidizes farmers who grow corn. This keeps the price of corn down. Cheap corn means cheap high-fructose corn syrup.

Cheap high-fructose corn syrup means food manufacturers can add sugar to just about any food, at an extremely small cost. I'm willing to guess that many of the foods you remember eating at your last meal have corn syrup in them, thanks to the U.S. government.

I've listed some of the more obvious influencers in your food choosing process, but it's even more complicated than this. Your emotional state can influence what and when you eat. Some people tend to eat more when they are depressed or stressed. Others eat according to the time of day rather than the sensation of hunger. Snacking has very little to do with actual hunger and more to do with mood, environment and access to food. Your decision on what to eat is actually determined by a whole host of influences, pressures, traditions and social manipulations carefully designed to help you make a certain choice. The one word that best describes all of these influences is culture. Culture is what we call our shared attitudes, values and the particular characteristics of the society in which we live.

Remember my friend Paul who struggles to control his weight? His earlier attempts to lose weight were successful because for a while he was able to withstand the various influences, traditions and manipulations that made him eat too much of the wrong kinds of foods. During his momentary weight loss phases he created a new culture for himself. He underwent a momentary cultural transformation by actively removing himself from the weight gaining lifestyle he typically enjoyed and instead paid attention to a set of new health-promoting cultural influences. For a while, he was able to better control all of the food choice influences that touched him every time he ate. Eventually, his daily choices and lifestyle slowly reverted to the same choices he was making during his weight gaining years.

Right now, most of us are drifting aimlessly in a sea of unhealthy influences unaware of or indifferent to the subtle pressures to eat certain foods or live a certain way. We are up to our necks in our western, unhealthy culture and most of us don't even know it. We're living our lives just like everybody else, swimming in the same cultural stew while our society slowly becomes the heaviest human population in world history.

The question as to why so many people are experiencing chronic diseases and gaining excessive body weight can be answered simply by watching the life of my neighbor Paul. His struggles with weight are caused by the culture in which he lives. When he changes that culture, he experiences some success in altering his weight. As soon as he reverts back to the old cultural norms, the weight returns. Admittedly, this is a pretty simplistic explanation to a very complex problem, but this simple analogy is actually profound. It helps us identify the real problem, the real reason so many people have chronic diseases and excessive body weight.

It has taken decades to create our current culture. Indeed, it has taken generations to assimilate our collective values and traditions and produce new ways of living that we now consider to be normal. Because the process of creating our current culture takes so long, we don't recognize changes as they occur, at least not until something bad happens. The poor health of Americans is one of those bad things that is a direct result of our culture.

In the 1970s when my mother was reacting to commercials to purchase Malt-O-Meal, my father was involved in sales. He would come home from long road trips and bring in the food he had purchased along the way. I loved seeing my dad, but even more, I loved the food he brought with him. While traveling the highways and byways of America he lived on junk food. His leftovers were my introduction to the world of fantastic tasting foods. I was able to taste Cheetos, Mystic Mint chocolate-mint cookies, Cheez Whiz, (cheese spread that comes in a can) and smoked meats and jerky. No one thought to question our food choices then. After all, we'd just sent men and rockets to the moon, microwave ovens were in every home and we acted with the swagger of the most powerful nation on earth. If a country as powerful as ours could harness the energy of the atom, we could easily create highly processed foods that taste great and contribute to the good health of all citizens. There was no reason to doubt that we had truly entered a new era in human nutrition. In actuality, it played out something like this:

- Highly processed food is delicious, inexpensive and since it was developed by scientists it must be good for you
- Processed and fast foods become common foods
- U.S. culture changes

Time passes…

- As new foods are invented they become normal foods (think Crisco, margarine, and high-fructose corn syrup)
- Chronic diseases like heart disease and diabetes start becoming more common, but no one knows why
- Obesity prevalence starts increasing, but no one knows why

Time passes…

- Studies start identifying unhealthy foods as possible causes
- Over time, the U.S. culture is dramatically different than it used to be
- Food manufacturers hire lobbyists and lawyers to fight any who oppose them
- FDA and dietitians are controlled by the food industry and turn a blind eye
- U.S. citizens have more obesity and chronic diseases than any other population and the cause of the problem is a mystery
- Businesses and government refuse to admit there is a problem or don't have the political will to change. Government doesn't want to hurt business or jobs, that's bad
- Culture is finally, reluctantly identified as the true culprit.

It takes decades of living in an unhealthy culture before any real, measurable side effects can be identified. Likewise, it has taken many years of research and critical thought to figure out why our health has gotten steadily worse. I'm not the first to claim that our unhealthy culture is the problem. Others have also connected the dots and have come to the same exact conclusions. We may have taken different paths along the way, but many of the best and brightest thinkers in health are now focused on two fundamental facts about our health.

1. **Our unhealthy behaviors and subsequent poor health are caused by the culture we have created.**
2. **The ONLY realistic solution to better health (including long term weight loss) is to change our culture.**

This is a good news/bad news/good news scenario. The first good news is that we are very confident that we have identified the real cause of our continued decline in health. The obesity epidemic, the diabetes epidemic and the majority of chronic diseases in the world today are caused by poor health behaviors that arise from our unhealthy culture. The bad news is that our culture is extremely difficult to alter. It took decades for our culture to become what it is today and it will likely take just as long to change it. The thought of trying to get multinational food conglomerates to stop producing unhealthy foods is enough to make me want to curl up and cry. Changing an entire culture is almost impossible to do, but to have a sustainable healthy lifestyle you don't have to change the whole culture, just your immediate environment that surrounds you. This is the remaining good news. Changing your immediate culture is achievable. People are successful with it all the time.

You all know someone who struggles with weight like Paul my neighbor. Most likely you also know people who do not struggle with weight, someone who has been able to withstand cultural pressure to live a healthy lifestyle. Somehow, despite the toxic culture we are all swimming in, they have been able to avoid the cultural influences that surround them. It's like they live on an island, removed from the culture that surrounds them. They are able to eat differently, exercise regularly and live a healthy lifestyle despite pressure to do otherwise. These island natives are important because they can show us how it's done—just like the 15% of weight loss study participants who were still successful after three years.

Culture Clash

We know that the cultural influences that surround us have resulted in an epidemic of obesity and chronic diseases. To reverse and prevent these unhealthy trends we will need to battle these cultural influences. Of course, I do want to point out that this book is not intended to promote some sort of counter culture revolution where we all forsake our modern conveniences and make a triumphant return to an ancient way of living. To be sure, the 21st century is here to stay—there is no turning back the clock and unwinding all that our modern society has created. Rather, we do have the option to pick and choose the aspects of our society that are truly beneficial—and that is exactly what the remainder of this book will focus on.

The idea of having a clash with our current culture is nothing new. In fact, we have experienced several culture conflicts throughout U.S. history. The issues and influences are slightly different, but the process to battle cultural influences has remained the same. The process goes like this: our culture undergoes subtle changes that continue to progress until unintended side effects appear that concern or endanger other people. The clash occurs when people begin to push back against the cultural tides. Take tobacco use for example. For the better part of 100 years smoking in the U.S. was extremely common. At one point over half of Americans smoked. Smoking was allowed in offices, schools, trains and even in airplanes. It was culturally acceptable to smoke at any time and in any location. As the dangers of tobacco use become more evident, people started to think about changing the status quo by fighting against the tobacco culture that permeated every aspect of our society.

To protect children and other family members, many smokers stopped smoking in their homes, preferring to light up outside. We set rules and laws to prohibit smoking from certain places and we set up designated smoking areas. Every time I pass the smoking area of the airport I feel terrible for all the smokers inside. It reminds me of how we isolate and treat animals in a zoo. But we do it to contain the exposure to smoke. Our clash with the tobacco culture has helped us create a society where non-smokers can be better protected from the harmful effects of smokers. Today people can eat, live and work without exposure to dangerous tobacco smoke. The battle to protect the public from the harmful effects of tobacco has taken almost a century and the battle is still raging. This example of a culture clash reminds us that change can happen, but it takes time—lots of it.

Culture clashes have happened in several other instances, including pollution regulations due to environmental destruction like the Cuyahoga River mentioned in the preface. The establishment of the movie rating system allows parents to have some control over the media content their children see. Today's movie rating system happened because individuals wanted some protections against the "all movies are good" movie culture. Today it is hard to imagine a time when automobiles did not have seat belts, but there was a time when a seat belt requirement was viewed as an intrusion on the personal right to use an automobile the way the owner wanted to. It was culturally acceptable and normal NOT to wear a seat belt. For a while, automobile manufacturers even refused to build cars with seat belts. That all began to change when more research started showing that seat belts saved and protected lives. The government finally got involved and the culture of seat belt free driving began to change. Today, you and I enjoy not only the benefits of added safety with a seat belt, but car manufacturers now routinely install airbags, antilock brakes and other safety enhancements, which are all part of a new "safety" culture.

Pushing back against the prevailing cultural tide is how we keep people protected from companies, organizations and sometimes even governments who have both a financial and political interest in making sure nothing upsets the status quo. At the very core of this cultural pressure is greed—the unrelenting pursuit of money, no matter what the cost, impact or collateral damage might be. More on this later.

Proof Points

I've mentioned this before, but I'm one of the most skeptical people I know. Before I believe what's said (or written) I usually have many questions. I like to gather as much evidence as I can for and against an issue before I give it my full attention. To me, evidence is the supportive material I need to be confident that what I'm learning is actually true. You should be equally skeptical of what I'm saying in this book, skeptical enough to ask questions and consider the evidence. After all, I'm not the first person to make such bold declarations about the solution to our weight and chronic disease issues, nor will I be the last. Every time I hear the news or browse the web or a magazine I see articles publicizing the latest discovery or solution to our poor health status.

Researchers may publish a paper showing that a particular gene is associated with diabetes or obesity. The media then spins the story to make it more appealing to a hungry viewer audience. The original research most likely stated that the findings were preliminary or that further testing is needed, but the media may hit you with a tantalizing title, "Research reveals the genetic cause for obesity." If it's not a story about the genetic connections to poor health we might blame the problem on nutrient deficiencies, toxins in the water or even hormonal imbalances due to menopause. Admittedly, all these solutions are way more exciting than the boring assertion that our culture is to blame, but hear me out. I think you might be more convinced after you see the large body of evidence that points directly to our culture as the culprit.

It's Not Just Us

Remember the obesity graph I showed in Chapter 1? It shows an astonishing upward trend in obesity in the U.S. The data used to create that graph only included American adults. Now look at this graph:

Past And Projected Overweight Rates In Selected Countries

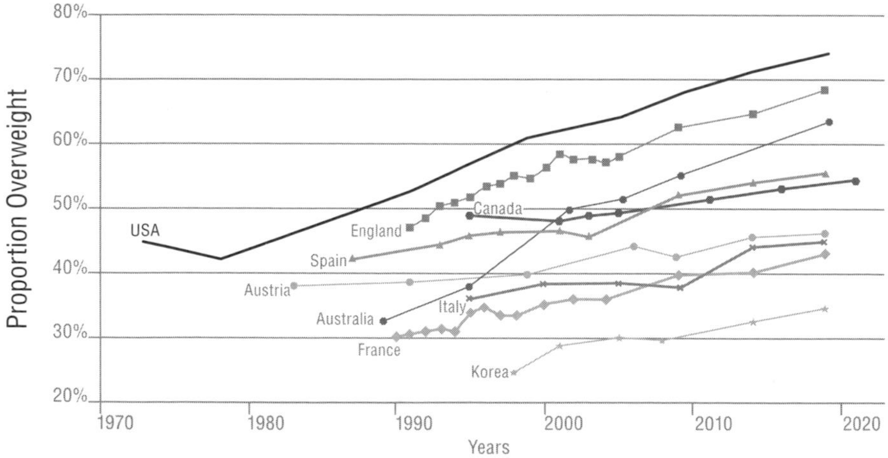

(² Adapted from Sassi, 2009)

It shows the percentage of people who are overweight or obese from a variety of countries. As mentioned earlier, the U.S. has the highest percentage of actual and predicted rates of overweight of all countries listed. However, this specific graph adds to our story. It shows that the increasing trend is not just an American health concern; the same increases are seen in all westernized countries. You may have heard that Asians and those who live around the Mediterranean are really healthy. That used to be true, but as these countries become westernized, we are seeing that their citizens are gaining excess weight and developing chronic diseases and are slowly losing their good health status. This graph tells much about the impact of our culture.

The trends for each country are essentially the same. They are all on a sustained upward trajectory which begs the question: What do all these countries have in common? Whatever it is, it appears that the U.S. started the trend. The citizens of these countries don't share the same genetic code, so that can't be it. Their citizens all live in different parts of the world, so they don't share the same environment, air or similar exposure to toxins. They do, however, share the same exposure to fast food, high calorie drinks, highly processed foods, fatty meats, dairy, cooking oils and few fruits and vegetables. Their food culture has changed in precisely the same way our food culture has changed. What they all have in common is the adoption of our western culture. Some have called this process globalization.

Globalization refers to the integration of global economies, the sharing of trade, business capital, labor markets and culture. The key word here is culture. As each of these countries becomes more globalized, they adopt many of the same food, beverage and eating traditions that are part of our American culture. Along with western business practices and free trade comes western food and western lifestyle. What this chart really shows is that residents of these countries are just like us, but some of them started a little later. They are beginning to struggle with exactly the same health issues you and I have. They struggle with diabetes, high blood pressure and cholesterol, and they struggle and fail miserably to reach and maintain a healthy body weight. In short, many nations are struggling with the same need to withstand assimilation into a western culture.

Besides having increasingly poor diets, people around the globe who live in industrialized countries are struggling to stay physically active. Computer technology, labor saving devices and transportation options have made it increasingly difficult to be physically active.[3] Lack of healthy food and opportunities for regular exercise are not an issue in poor countries of the world, rather only countries that have become westernized are struggling to maintain healthy lifestyles.

This data also hints that some countries are struggling more than others. Because most of us live in the U.S. it's hardest for us to notice the changes that are occurring to ourselves, but we've changed the most because our culture has changed the most.

Not long ago I was entertaining colleagues from South America. As my friends arrived in Atlanta's international airport, they were stunned to see so many large, overweight people. This shock was repeated as they traveled around the U.S. noticing the size of Americans. Eventually, we had some time to visit and I asked them what surprised them most about America. Unanimously they all mentioned that they were stunned to see how big (fat) Americans were. I was not surprised by their response because compared to their own citizens, Americans are much larger. In America's defense, I was quick to mention that only 21% of Americans smoke, compared to their 49%, but my retort fell on deaf ears. They didn't want to hear about smoking rates; they now had evidence to confirm what they heard, but never quite believed. America has the heaviest population in the world.

Worse Than You Know

One day I was reading one of the scientific health journals and I read this sincere plea from the article's authors, "application of these nutrition and exercise guidelines will help curb the rising epidemics of obesity, metabolic syndrome, hypertension, diabetes and cardiovascular disease." I can relate to these authors' attempts to encourage a healthier lifestyle and I wondered what segment of the U.S. population the authors had studied. I was shocked to learn that this study was from India.[4] This wasn't Orlando, Memphis, or Pittsburgh, this was a plea for healthier lifestyles going out to the residents of Calcutta, New Delhi, and Bangalore—faraway places with drastically different societies, all suffering from the same lifestyle-caused epidemics that we are.

Increased rates of obesity and chronic diseases are happening all over the world. As people abandon their traditional culture and lifestyle in favor of a western lifestyle, the diseases that are associated with the new culture begin to afflict the population. In Canada, the highest rates of obesity and diabetes are found among the Canadian Arctic Inuit.[5] Our western culture knows no bounds—it now stretches around the globe and as far north as the Arctic. Here is the list of countries that have the highest rates of diabetes.

Ranking	Country	Cases of Diabetes (in millions)
1	India*	31.7
2	China*	20.8
3	U.S.*	17.0
4	Indonesia	8.4
5	Japan*	6.8
6	Pakistan	5.2
7	Russian Federation	4.6
8	Brazil*	4.6
9	Italy*	4.3
10	Bangladesh	3.2

([6]Adapted from Wild, 2004)

There is no question that our western culture now impacts most countries in the world.[7] Some countries are worse than others because some countries have been more aggressive to adopt a western lifestyle. Think of the countries that have openly embraced and practice capitalism. I think of countries that have economies that are quickly catching up with America. If you look at the 10 largest economies in the world, six of them also have the highest number of diabetes cases. Countries that produce lots of goods and services have more of a western culture. They also have more obesity, diabetes and chronic diseases.

Besides the largest economies, you can also look at countries with the fastest growing economies, where westernization is happening at a faster pace. In these countries, you'll also find the fastest increases in diabetes. Westernization is happening at a rapid rate in Egypt, Jordan, Turkey, Indonesia, Qatar and Argentina. Not surprisingly, these same countries are also seeing some of the fastest increases in obesity and diabetes. Dr. Darwiche, the head of the Rashid Center for Diabetes in the United Arab Emirates, describes the new culture this way, "It is actually cheaper to eat fast food than to cook healthy food at home. There is now an over-representation of cheap fast food in the region which is driving our diabetes epidemic."[8] Dr. Darwiche might as well be talking about Omaha, Nebraska or any other major U.S. city as he describes the causes of obesity and diabetes he is seeing in the Middle East.

Where westernization has taken hold the culture changes and this is especially true in urban settings. Urban communities are generally more progressive and quicker to adopt western ways than rural communities, and as such, highly processed and fast foods are more available in urban settings. If our western culture is really to blame for poor health we should see some evidence that as people move from rural to urban settings, they get greater exposure to an unhealthy culture. Researchers have looked at this very question.[9] Regardless of what country you consider, as people move from rural to urban settings food and physical activity habits change. With these changes, blood glucose, blood pressure and cholesterol levels increase. Rapid increases in diabetes and other chronic diseases are occurring in all westernized countries, but more particularly in many of the larger cities.

A Full Dose

There is yet another way to test the idea that our culture is to blame for our poor health. When doctors estimate health risks caused by tobacco smoke, they consider two factors: the exposure rate and the length of exposure. This is simply the number of cigarettes you smoke per day (rate) and how long you've smoked. Smokers' risk of chronic disease and early death can be accurately predicted by determining how many cigarettes they smoke combined with how long they've smoked. In the same way tobacco smoke exposure is linked to many chronic diseases and death, consuming a western diet and living a western lifestyle likewise increases your risk of chronic diseases and early death. Just like tobacco exposure, your exposure to western culture is linked to increased risks of chronic diseases and early death. Your risk of chronic disease can be determined by both the dose of your exposure to an unhealthy culture and the length of your exposure. For example, I try really hard to eat a healthy diet and stay physically active, despite pressure to do otherwise and I've been doing this for most of my life. My exposure to our unhealthy culture has been low. However, my son who is 15 years old is a typical teenager. His favorite food groups are the sugar group, the syrup group, the meat group and the ice cream group. His exposure to our western food culture is very high. Luckily, he's only been this way for a short while and I pray each day that he'll listen to his old man and start eating better. I'm hopeful that he'll soon improve his nutrition and exercise habits, thus keeping his exposure to our unhealthy culture as short as possible.

When you consider western culture as if it were like tobacco smoke or radiation you can then study how it impacts people. The comparison between the diet and lifestyle of my son and I is one example of how a different exposure rate might be studied. An even better comparison can be made when we look at those who migrate to the U.S. Consider a typical female who migrates from rural Mexico to the U.S. The culture she left is a traditional, rural, Latin lifestyle with traditional foods and cooking behaviors. Compared to our U.S. diet patterns, she is in the habit of eating less saturated fat, sugar and junk food and more corn tortillas.[10] Her traditional Mexican culture is actually healthier than the one she encounters in the U.S. When she arrives in her new country she is suddenly confronted with U.S. food culture, which may have very little in common with the foods from her native land. In the beginning, the rate of exposure and the length of the exposure are low because she just arrived, but with time, she will change. Within one generation (about 22 years) she will have lost almost all of her Mexican dietary habits and culture; she will have become westernized, just like the rest of us.[10]

Immigrant exposure to our American culture intensifies the longer they are here. When new immigrants arrive in the U.S. they weigh considerably less than U.S.-born residents. Their BMI scores are two to five percent lower. But after 10 to 15 years, new immigrants and U.S.-born residents weigh just as much if not more than the American average.[11] Another study compared the rate of obesity between new immigrants (those who had been in the U.S. for less than one year) and immigrants who had been in the U.S. for 15 years or longer. New immigrants had an obesity rate of eight percent compared to 19% for the immigrants who had been in the U.S. longer.[12] The only difference between the two groups is how long they'd been in the U.S. and more specifically, how long they'd been exposed to our culture.

When immigrants move from one country to the next they gradually begin to accept and live according to the cultural norms of the new country. Dietary acculturation is the name scientists use to describe the act of slowly assimilating into the new country's food culture.[13] If the new diet includes westernized food, obesity and chronic diseases begin to take hold. But this can also work in reverse. I've had family members who left the U.S. to do humanitarian service in rural Uganda. In essence, they migrated from a typical western American culture to an agrarian, rural, African culture. There is no fast or processed food in that part of the world; they only eat what they can grow locally. Not surprisingly, these members of my family lost weight and quickly saw improvements in blood cholesterol, blood pressure and glucose after just a few short months of being acculturated in to a healthier way of living.

More than any other piece of evidence, studies of immigrant health and nutrition present the clearest proof that our culture is to blame for our poor health. Studies of native Japanese and Japanese-Americans show that the high rates of cardiovascular disease in the United States are directly related to our American lifestyle. The connection between heart disease and American culture becomes very clear when you begin to follow rates of heart disease among Japanese citizens who live in Japan, and Japanese citizens who have migrated to Hawaii and California. Native Japanese had almost no cases of heart disease, while disease rates among Japanese men in Hawaii were dramatically greater than those in Japan, and those who had migrated to California had 50% more heart disease than those in Hawaii. Blood cholesterol levels and blood glucose levels also increased with increased exposure to American culture.[14] The cause of heart disease is obviously related to the degree to which the immigrants adopted the American lifestyle. These results cannot be caused by genetics because the changes in heart disease rates occurred within one generation.

There is also a direct relationship between the length of time immigrants are in the U.S. and how much body fat they have. It doesn't matter which country immigrants come from or how old they are, (children, adolescents, adults) the longer they are here the more they weigh.[15–16]

As mentioned earlier, the U.S. isn't the only country to have an unhealthy culture. Any time an immigrant migrates from a country that is less westernized to one that is more westernized, dietary acculturation occurs. When it happens in the U.S. the results are more obvious because we offer a much stronger dose of an unhealthy culture than other countries. When Chinese immigrants migrated to Hong Kong, Taiwan, Singapore, Western Europe or the U.S. their rates of cardiovascular disease increased substantially, despite having similar medication use.[17] In another study, women who migrated from Punjabi India to Vienna Austria were compared to women still living in Punjabi. Those who had immigrated were two to three times more likely to be obese, once again showing that acculturation is to blame for the worsening of immigrant health.[18] When people move from a healthy culture to an unhealthy western culture they adopt new behaviors that lead to chronic disease and early death.

Louisiana Culture Clash

I live in the Rocky Mountains. Recently, I spent several weeks working for a mining company in Louisiana. During the weeks I was there I had the privilege of eating with the employees. Now I agree that this is not the same as a country to country migration, and a two week stay hardly makes me an immigrant, but the experience shows how the dietary acculturation process can happen even within the U.S. Besides, my trip might as well be treated just like a migration because the only thing I had in common with these workers was use of the English language and even that could be debated.

In the few weeks I was there I had fried catfish, fried shrimp, fried chicken, fried hushpuppies, fried okra, chicken gumbo, sausage gumbo, shrimp gumbo, fish gumbo, mystery gumbo, barbequed spare ribs, barbequed beans, barbequed chicken, barbequed pork, something that resembled coleslaw, and a dish that consisted of chicken wrapped in bacon, dipped in cheese. Every breakfast consisted of biscuits and gravy, sausage, bacon, ham, eggs, and a variety of flat foods (French toast, waffles, pancakes) made from refined white flour. Every once in a while I could find a glass of juice or a lonely piece of fruit. I was being rapidly acculturated (seduced) into a dramatically different way of eating and the longer I stayed, the more my food shock was being replaced with food acceptance and the more I became accustomed to their way of eating.

I was fortunate to escape without any arterial damage or a sudden stroke, but my bowels took some time to recover. During this two week period, I received a concentrated dose of new culture. Luckily the length of my exposure was brief. These miners are the backbone of America, men and women who work hard jobs, live hard lives and are doing their best to support their families. Their daily diet reflects cultural influences that run deep throughout the south. My friends in Louisiana eat the same way their parents did and for most of them, there is absolutely nothing wrong with their food and exercise culture. But there is no question that continued exposure to that lifestyle will eventually take a drastic toll on health.

Why We Like The New Culture

When our culture changes, we generally change with it because we don't always have an option. When I was in Louisiana, my options were to eat with the local workers or go hungry. This is the same thing that happens to our kids at school—they eat what is served in the cafeteria. This also happens with every vending machine. Your snacking options were determined by someone else. You can make a selection from the choices placed before you or you can go without. Our culture dictates what foods are popular and we eat what's available to us. There is another reason we eat according to our culture. Popular food choices are generally delicious tasting foods that are relatively inexpensive and extremely convenient. The taste, cost and convenience of foods are maximized in our western culture. Our daily food selections have moved away from foods that take a long time to prepare to foods that are fast and simple to make. Today's popular foods are fast, simple meals that taste good. Pizza delivery is fast and simple, that's why it is so popular. All you need is some money and a phone and you don't even have to get up.

We've embraced our new culture and it's even viewed with envy by others. When asked what they liked most about America, a couple of my European friends were quick to list doughnuts, maple bars and cinnamon rolls—yummy foods made with lots of fat, sugar and salt. They liked the way they tasted. They also liked chips, tacos, hot dogs, pepperoni pizza, waffles, French fries and ice cream. After tasting these and other foods they were beginning to understand why Americans were so big. They envy the delicious food, but not the diseases that go along with it.

Sometimes immigrants to the U.S. are quick to adopt our new culture because they feel pressure to be westernized. They are under extreme pressure to learn English, get jobs and support their families. Many have preconceived ideas of what being an American is like and many of them want to experience everything America has to offer, including our fast, processed foods. Individuals who want to quickly assimilate our American culture find that consuming American food is one of the fastest ways to be seen as authentically American.[19] Every American meal they consume contains an additional 182 calories and 12 extra grams of fat compared to their traditional meals. Acculturation among immigrants occurs because these new arrivals want to be American. As I've said before, "if you want to live like an American, you will die like an American."

The changes in the taste of our westernized food were not caused by accidentally discovering different combinations of food flavors and textures. The popular foods we eat today are actually the product of decades of careful manipulation of three basic ingredients: fat, sugar and salt. The food industry has been acutely aware of the nuances of human taste and appetite and has created foods that are better aligned with our taste preferences. Today, our food culture is nothing more than the outcome of decades of food manipulation.

The food industry has developed foods that Americans love to eat and as these foods have become more popular they have become mainstays of our food culture. Decades of exposure to this culture is now producing the unfortunate side effects of obesity, diabetes and other chronic diseases.

I have suggested that the real cause of our poor health is our unhealthy culture. I've tried to demonstrate how worsening health in all westernized countries is proof that culture is to blame. Studies of the health of immigrants also support this explanation. If our poor health is really caused by our unhealthy culture, why haven't organizations and governments done something to help improve the culture? As you are about to learn there are several good reasons why they haven't done, and most likely won't do, much to stop it.

Island Native

My name is Stacey and I live in Baltimore where I work as an events coordinator. I have always had a hard time maintaining a healthy weight, and as I got older I noticed that my weight was making it harder for me to get around. The reality of living an unhealthy lifestyle really hit home for me when my husband was diagnosed with pre-diabetes and a fatty liver due to his unhealthy lifestyle. I knew that it was time for a change if my husband and I were going to be healthy and free of disease.

In order to reverse the effects of my bad lifestyle, I began with a simple choice to drink more water. Simple was the focus in most of my choices. I drank water instead of soda, juice or milk. My meals included more lean cuts of meat, more fruits and vegetables and to top it off I just tried to eat smaller servings. These may not seem like much, but my family and I have always eaten unhealthy foods. I made small changes to my diet that were simple and sustainable. After a while of eating healthy, I realized that I needed to get more exercise in my life.

I don't like exercising so staying committed to regular exercise has never been easy for me. Luckily, my employer offers several exercise classes at work. I participate in their strength training, cycling, and I really like the Zumba classes. I know that finding the exercise classes I like has played a key part in getting more exercise.

Even though I was incorporating simple changes into my life, I still needed help to remain successful. I had to get some help from my cousin in order to stay motivated. My cousin had made big changes in her life before I did and she really helped me stay motivated by telling me what she did. It was also very helpful to have friends on Facebook tell me how proud they were and encourage me to keep it up. My husband helped me stay motivated by challenging me to participate in a weight loss competition. These changes haven't been easy for me because it has required that I do things differently and that's hard because I don't like change. If I had one bit of advice I would tell people to reach out to a spouse or friend who will support and change with you. It's easier to have new food and exercise habits when you have someone supporting you.

CHAPTER 4

Buy, Taste, Crave, Repeat

LET'S TAKE A QUIZ. IGNORE WHAT YOU'VE LEARNED ABOUT HEALTHY FOODS SO FAR AND THINK ABOUT A FOOD YOU CRAVE. I'M NOT TALKING ABOUT YOUR FAVORITE HEALTHY FOOD, I WANT YOU TO THINK ABOUT A FOOD YOU ABSOLUTELY LOVE. Have you got one in mind? Now answer this question: Which of the following three ingredients are in the food you selected: salt, sugar or fat? One food I often crave is bacon. Normal bacon has salt and fat, the combination of which makes it delicious, but I've also seen honey or maple-glazed bacon which includes salt, sugar and fat which makes it even more delicious.

You may have selected a food loaded with fat and sugar like chocolate, cheesecake, ice cream, doughnuts, brownies or a milk shake. Or maybe you selected foods with heaping doses of salt and fat like pizza, popcorn, bacon, pretzels, bread sticks, cheese, French Fries, hot dogs, sausage or gravy. Perhaps the food you crave the most contains a trifecta of flavors, a combination of all three ingredients combined in a way that makes them irresistible. These could include McDonald's sausage, egg and cheese McGriddle, Denny's banana caramel French toast skillet or Dairy Queen's peanut buster parfait.

I'm willing to bet that almost all of you have selected a food that has at least two of these three ingredients. In the quiz, I was careful to ask for foods that you crave, not just want or like, but really desire. I did this because I wanted you to reach into your brain and think about the foods that have really had an impact on you, foods that bring back memories, smells and emotions that are pleasurable to you. Foods that you crave today are foods that when eaten in the past caused you to have an emotional response that was carefully recorded by your brain. You associate the food as a pleasurable experience because the food actually helped create a pleasurable experience.

Your Ancient Taste Buds

To really understand why we struggle to eat healthy foods, we need to understand how our food can have such a powerful influence over us. For a moment, let's revisit our ancient ancestors. They lived in a time when there was little if any access to salt, sugar and fat. For almost all of human history salt was a very rare commodity. Even the ancient Roman civilization did not have access to much salt. It was so scarce that it was treated just like gold or silver. In fact Roman soldiers were often paid in salt, which was used by the soldiers to trade for other foods and goods. The word "salary" is a derivative from the Latin salārium or salt money. Not until the modern industrial age did salt become available to the masses. Today, salt is so plentiful that we dump it on roads in the winter to keep them from freezing. All animals require a certain amount of salt to function properly and our bodies have about the same salt content as the oceans, but historically the salt in our bodies came naturally from the foods we ate. Even though those foods don't contain much salt, they contain enough to keep us healthy. It would have been impossible to salt our food or add salt to anything because there was no naturally occurring salt for most humans. Humans never got accustomed to the taste of salt because it simply was not available. Many of us crave the taste of salt because according to our ancient bodies, we've never had it before. It's a new taste sensation to our ancient taste buds. When we taste salt, our taste buds tell our brains that whatever this is we like it and we want more of it. Today, we have salt shakers because we like the taste of salt so much. Of course, taste alone doesn't fully explain why we like salt so much.

When we eat something, feel something or do something pleasurable our brains release neurochemicals that are associated with pleasure. With these chemicals, we get a pleasurable sensation, a rush of feeling good. Certain parts of our brains are actually responsible for detecting and recognizing pleasurable experiences. We like the taste of salt, but we also crave salt and when we eat it part of our brain gets activated and we sense a certain amount of pleasure. It may not always be obvious, but if a salty food provides a certain amount of pleasure our brains will remember that salty food was the source of that pleasure. Because of this pleasure sensation, our brains will encourage us to consume salt again. Some have suggested that the desire for salt can actually evolve into a subtle addiction.[1] For 100,000 years humans did not have access to salt. When we eat it today, we like it so much that we are willing to add extra salt to our food and purchase foods that contain lots of salt.

Sugar was another ingredient that was unavailable to humans for almost all of human history. There are three basic types of sugars: sugar found in milk called galactose, the type of sugar used by our cells called glucose and the sugar that is found naturally in plants called fructose. All other sugars are just different combinations of these three. For example, table sugar is glucose and fructose combined. Compare the taste of a fresh peach with the taste of a teaspoon of table sugar. Both have a sweet sensation, but they don't taste quite the same; they are chemically slightly different. Which of these three basic sugars did our ancient ancestors have access to? Well, they had galactose from milk as infants while they were nursing, but for most of their lives they did not have access to milk.

The only sugar they had access to was fructose and only during short periods of time. I have a fruit orchard in my garden. Each fall my family helps me harvest cherries, raspberries, peaches, pears, apples, apricots, plums, nectarines and grapes. If we don't bottle them or preserve them within just a few days the fruit spoils. Every fall for 100,000 years our ancestors did the same thing, but they did not have the ability to preserve the fruit, so they stuffed themselves with as much fruit as they could eat. Much of the fructose in these fruits was converted to fat and stored in the body. The fat would then be used to keep them alive during the winter when food was scarce. Our ancient ancestors ate fructose in its natural form, in limited amounts and only for a very limited time. Outside of fall harvest, there was no fructose. White table sugar wasn't available for consumption until the late 1800s. Today, sugar, especially fructose, is not just available at the fall fruit harvest, it's available at Halloween, Thanksgiving, Christmas, Valentine's Day, Easter and at every other holiday of the year. Sugar is available everywhere at any time and just like our ancestors, we gorge ourselves and the sugar is stored as extra fat in anticipation of a foodless winter that never arrives. After decades of year-round sugar harvesting we've become the fattest population on the planet. Rather than eat a peach, we consume a six pack of Dr. Pepper. Both have fructose, but one comes from the earth for a very limited amount of time while the other is available 24 hours a day, seven days a week. One comes with fiber and an array of health-promoting phytochemicals while the other comes with 23 secret ingredients.

Our preference for the taste and pleasure that comes from sugar is even more powerful than our desire for salt. Parents often use the word "addiction" to describe a child's habit of binging on sugar and craving more. Children and adults do seem to show strong desires for foods that contain sugar. The pleasure that comes from eating sugary foods has been well documented and some have suggested that our unhealthy cravings for foods made from sugar are not unlike other addictions.[2] Addiction may still be too strong a word for our relationship to sugar, but there is certainly a very, very strong attraction. Americans are not alone in their attraction to sugar. In 2011, U.S. farmers exported almost 600,000 metric tons of high-fructose corn syrup to other nations so they can fulfill the same cravings (or addictions?) we possess for sugar.

If salt was nonexistent in the ancient world and fructose was only available for a limited time, then the limited consumption of fats by our ancient relatives is no different. As we discussed earlier, our ancestors ate meat and some of that meat likely had a limited amount of animal fat associated with it. Outside of occasional animal fat, there were no vegetable oils, butter, margarine, Crisco or processed oils of any kind. Fried foods are a product of the industrial age, not the Stone Age, which means ranch dressing, French fries, doughnuts, fried chicken, and Chili's Texas Cheese Fries with its 2,200 calories were nonexistent for all of ancient humanity. Our ancestors never tasted the creamy texture and subtle melting that we sense when we eat fried catfish or hot French fries because they never had the oils needed to cook them. Just like salt and sugar, the taste and texture of foods cooked in added fats and oils are relatively unknown to our ancient taste buds, so when we taste our high fat foods, we get an instant pleasurable sensation; the experience gets recorded in our brains and we look for opportunities to do it again. Like our first taste of ice cream, it doesn't take much to get our brains to quickly recognize that certain foods can cause a pleasurable reaction that is not soon forgotten.

Our ancient bodies are stuck in time; they are not accustomed to tasting salt, sugar and fat individually, and when they do, the pleasure centers in our brains light up. When these three flavors are combined, the pleasure experience is amplified even more. As tasty and addictive as these three ingredients can be by themselves, something magical happens when they are combined. Our brains are overwhelmed by the taste experience, the event is carefully recorded in our memories and if the opportunity to repeat the experience ever comes around again, our brain will do its best to remind us how good it was by releasing a craving—an intense desire to do it again. Each time we give into a craving we close the loop on what food scientists call "conditioned overeating." This is exactly why food manufacturers have been manipulating our food. They know that the carefully engineered combination of salt, sugar and fat stimulates the senses and creates subtle cravings that fuel our desire to keep buying. I call this process buy, taste, crave, repeat.

Maximizing Our Cravings

In 1987, Warren Buffett, one of the world's richest men famously stated, "I'll tell you why I like the cigarette business. It costs a penny to make. Sell it for a dollar. It's addictive. And there's fantastic brand loyalty." One of the most profitable industries in the world is the tobacco industry. Because smokers get addicted to the product, they become repeat customers who purchase on a regular basis. In many ways the food industry is just like the tobacco industry. The tobacco industry has carefully formulated their tobacco with chemicals that offer a delicate balance between creating an enjoyable smoking experience with a nicotine addiction that is just severe enough to keep smokers coming back for more. The food industry has also spent enormous time and resources creating highly processed foods that are so delicious that consumers will consistently purchase products over long periods of time. No one knows this better than Warren Buffet. Companies like Kraft Foods, Nestle, Coca-Cola, See's Candies, Dairy Queen and Outback Steakhouse are some of the world's best manipulators of food and each of them is entirely or partially owned by Warren Buffet.

Careful manipulation of fat, salt and sugar in the foods we eat has been a boon to food manufacturers; the holy grail of gaining repeat customers. And believe it or not, all of it is based on the emotional reaction our ancient bodies have to these delicious foods. In the early twentieth century, food manufacturers began noticing trends in how well different foods were selling. Over time it was discovered that foods with different amounts of fat, salt and sugar sold better than foods that did not contain these ingredients. It is interesting that fat, salt and sugar by themselves do not have the same appeal as when they are carefully blended. Which would you rather eat: 10 teaspoons of white sugar or a 12-ounce can of soda? Most of you would prefer the soda, even though it too contains 10 teaspoons of sugar. This is because sugar by itself is not a highly palatable food; only when it is carefully combined with other ingredients does it give us the kick we like so much. This same phenomenon is also true for fats and salt. By themselves, they have little appeal, but when carefully combined with each other an entire new eating experience is created.

My son came home from high school the other day with a new tag hanging on his key chain. The tag was a small plastic card in the shape of a miniature Wendy's chocolate shake called a Frosty. Wendy's knows that their sugar and fat-laden chocolate shakes are delicious. They also know that teenagers are regular customers. Anyone possessing the $1 plastic tag gets a free chocolate Frosty with any food or drink purchase. Wendy's has leveraged our instinctive cravings for sugar and fat into a successful customer loyalty program.

To do this, companies like Wendy's hire food scientists to help them create foods that offer the perfect blend of the three magic ingredients: salt, sugar and fat. The scientists know how much we like these ingredients because they are well aware of the different studies showing that foods with the three flavors are preferred by consumers. For example, researchers asked people to carefully record the different foods they ate over a seven-day period.[3] Once the meals were recorded they asked them to rate their preference for the foods on a scale of 1-7. Foods with the highest preferences were mostly foods with the most sugar and fat and when the amount of food eaten was considered, foods with the highest preferences were eaten in much higher quantities. If you want to sell more food, carefully create foods with higher amounts of sugar and fat.

Food engineers did not invent the chocolate chip cookie, but the cookie does illustrate how careful food design that uses salt, sugar and fat can create an emotional eating experience. Careful observation of a person eating a chocolate chip cookie reveals how the right ingredients combined with the right temperature and texture can produce a memorable eating event. My wife likes to improve the experience by adding oatmeal to the dough. The oatmeal gives the cookies a chewy texture. Fat from the butter is mixed with the chocolate and both melt at body temperature in a way that we actually feel the cookie change from a solid to a liquid state while it's being chewed. Salt from the butter satisfies our cravings for sodium and the sugar brings it all together in a delicious, melting, sweet and salty flavor extravaganza. This experience is even more enjoyable when the cookies are still warm from the oven. Somehow the warmer temperature enhances how the mouth experiences chewing and swallowing.

Not long ago, I was on one of my many speaking engagements when I had one of my less enjoyable travel experiences. I had just finished a very long flight, which had been delayed by bad weather. I was stuck in the middle seat between a fussy baby and someone who didn't smell too good. I was sleepy and a bit frazzled because of the long day of travel. When I arrived at the hotel front desk to check in, I could instantly smell hot chocolate chip cookies, which were sitting on a large platter right in front of me. The hotel employee offered me one, which I gladly accepted. While he processed my reservation I ate the cookie. All the stress and hassle I had experienced in my day of travel instantly melted away as I slowly chewed the delicious cookie. Its impact on me was like an instant sedative. My heart rate dropped to a normal range, my body felt warmer and all the stress and anxiety of my day melted away. A day or so later I was still staying in the same hotel and in the evening as I walked past the registration desk I had only one question on my mind, "I wonder if they have any more of those delicious chocolate chip cookies?" I was hoping to repeat the cookie-based healing experience I had encountered earlier.

Chocolate chip cookies are a great example of how all three ingredients can work together. Each cookie has salt and fat from the butter, sugar and fat from the chocolate chips and more sweetness from the added sugar. This cookie is deliberately designed to maximize our response to these three flavors. The effect of all three flavors blended together is so powerful that we often combine the three flavors without even realizing it. For example, suppose you decide to order pizza. Pizza is a classic example of a food high in salt and fat. Your pizza arrives and as you get ready to eat it, you grab a drink. What do you think is the number one beverage choice to go along with pizza? Here's a hint, think of something that can make salt and fat even more delicious. The most favorite beverage with salty and fatty pizza is soda. A 12-ounce can has 10 teaspoons of sugar. When we get ready to eat a pizza we automatically think about what we'd like as a beverage and almost without thinking we choose soda. The fructose in the soda elevates the two-flavored pizza to another level of deliciousness. Most of us will do exactly the same thing when we eat French fries. As good as hot French fries are (loaded with salt and fat) we once again elevate the experience by dipping the fries in sugar. We don't actually use real sugar, we use a sugar substitute called catsup. Catsup contains high-fructose corn syrup, corn syrup and salt. Our taste preferences know that the sugary taste of catsup makes our French fries even better. Almost subconsciously, we strive to arrange our food flavors so that we can get as close to taste perfection as possible.

Flavor Adoration

Whether it is the flavor of chocolate, ice cream, pizza, hot dogs, hamburgers, cupcakes, pies, or deep fried Twinkies, we have created a culture that not only supports foods with these three flavors, but actually expands their availability into every possible corner of society. This happens with many of our most favorite foods, but just for the sake of argument let's talk about how just one of these foods has managed to become an item of such adoration. Consider the ubiquitous pig part we all call bacon. Its ability to create an emotional response has helped bacon become a pervasive ingredient in all kinds of foods and celebrations.

- The cable channel The Food Network has a new food program called "Crave." In the show, the host travels around the country tasting popular tasty foods like barbeque, hamburgers, cheese burgers, pizza, fried chicken, fried cheese, chocolate and ice cream. The show is back by popular demand in its second season, and most of the foods characterized on the show contain bacon.
- Every year 3,000 Chicago residents pay $75 each to attend Baconfest Chicago where they can stuff themselves with foods made with bacon.
- New York City has the Bourbon and Bacon Expo.
- Des Moines, Iowa has the Blue Ribbon Bacon Festival which sells out with 4,500 attendees each year.
- Knoxville, Tennessee has their annual BaconFest.
- Keystone, Colorado has the Blue Ribbon Bacon Tour.
- Sacramento, California has the Sacramento Bacon Festival.
- Portland, Oregon has Baconfest.
- The Carvers Hamburger chain has giant billboards in major cities that have one simple message: Carvers: Shakes and Bacon.
- Boston, Massachusetts has the Boston Bacon and Beer Festival.
- Denny's restaurant has a bacon celebration called "Baconalia" that serves seven new bacon infused meals every day for 10 days. One of the more popular bacon foods is their maple bacon ice cream.

As much as I like bacon, others worship it. Bacon is big business because people love it. On average, every man, woman and child in the U.S. eats 18 pounds of bacon a year. A few years ago I spoke to a group of insurance professionals at a meeting in Missouri. This meeting was a bit unusual because it was being hosted at a fancy mountain resort and my only food options were to join the group for the three meals of the day. For the first time in my life I was served bacon for breakfast, lunch and dinner. Resorts aren't the only food providers serving up bacon.

Burger King has recently rolled out a new fresh-and-healthy food called California Whopper. It's a new hamburger covered with Swiss cheese and bacon, and I'm guessing they think it's now a healthy item because they've added guacamole. I can't help but wonder that if Burger King is coming out with a new line of foods called fresh-and-healthy, what does that say about their current food line up? Not so fresh-and-healthy? Fast food chain Sonic is adding three new breakfast burritos to its menu, including the Ultimate Meat & Cheese Breakfast Burrito, which contains sausage, bacon, tater tots, cheese sauce, cheddar cheese and eggs wrapped in a flour tortilla. KFC Canada has debuted its best-selling sandwich: the Double Down Bunless Chicken Sandwich. It includes two pieces of seasoned chicken, two pieces of processed pepper jack cheese and of course two pieces of bacon. Denny's vice president of marketing announced that Denny's will "answer the bacon appetites of the nation" with its new Maple Bacon Sundae, sprinkled with hickory-smoked bacon. (**www.meatpoultry.com**) Not to be outdone, Jack-in-the-Box also now has bacon flavored shakes.

A Complete Indulgence

This food experimentation and creativity isn't limited to just bacon. Food scientists are constantly striving to develop new foods that will leave customers craving more. As one food scientist put it, "the food industry is the master manipulator of your mind and desires." No doubt that you have already succumbed to this manipulation. It comes in the form of our desires for a Snickers bar, Oreo cookies, M&Ms, Cadbury Eggs, Krispy Kreme doughnuts, Kit-Kat chocolate bars and even Starbucks coffee. Yes, just when you thought I was done poking holes in all of your favorite foods I still had to mention your breakfast cup of coffee. Coffee is not the problem, it only becomes a real issue when your coffee experience gets elevated with added fat and sugar, like when you order a Double Chocolate Chip Frappuccino Blended Crème with whipped cream that has 600 calories and is packed with delicious fat, sugar and yes, salt. No wonder it does such a great job of waking people up in the morning!

Food scientists understand why we like what we like. They understand the complex dance that takes place between our taste buds and smell receptors, and when we chew and swallow our food. They know that food textures and layers used in different ways can enhance the eating experience. Snickers, Kit-Kat and M&Ms are deliciously layered treats that melt at precisely the temperature found in your mouth. When a food has been caramelized, it has been coated with a thin coating of caramel, a layer of sugar and fat. The sensation of chewing through the layers and the tastes of salt, sugar and fat make for a rewarding experience.

If you've traveled through an airport lately you've been manipulated by the master food manipulator that is Cinnabon®. Cinnabon is a fast food chain that makes cinnamon rolls. At Cinnabon, there is no reason for aggressive advertising because all they need to do is pump the aroma of baking cinnamon rolls out into the air. The smell alone can elicit an emotional reaction and can cause us to immediately purchase a tasty roll. With Cinnabon, it's all about the eating experience. After years of careful culinary creating, Cinnabon has perfected the flavor, layer and texture combination. The Cinnabon Classic Cinnamon Roll has 36 grams of fat, 17 of which are saturated. That's almost a full day's worth of saturated fat in one roll. It contains 56 grams of sugar—a can of Pepsi has 41 grams. It also contains 830 milligrams of sodium making it a salt, sugar and fat masterpiece. But perfection is not reached until the dough is carefully rolled and baked so that the outside layers are chewier than the inside layers—all of which are covered by a creamy frosting. Finally, the entire thing is served hot. When I think about this creation I'm reminded of Warren Buffet again who likes the idea of investing in products that are addictive. Foods that fuel our desires manipulate our purchasing habits. Fortunes are built on this principle.

Waffles, a Chicago-based waffle company, also understands our cravings well. Their company motto is, "A complete indulgence in sweet and savory delights." Sports bars in Texas serve chicken wrapped in bacon, dipped in cheese because it stimulates our taste senses and because it sells well.

The number one source of salt in the American diet is not from chips or fast foods—it's bread. Sandwich bread, buns, rolls and muffins contain fairly large amounts of sodium. Since we eat a lot of bread, we also get a lot of sodium. No doubt the added salt makes us eat more of it because we like the taste.

I've already admitted my partiality toward salty and fatty foods. I don't think my fondness rises to the level of obsession. I do like these foods, but they don't exert much influence over my food choices. For me, Cinnabon with its culinary perfection is not a temptation. In fact, I don't have a strong attraction toward ice cream, chocolate and a lot of other foods that many people find hard to resist. My wife thinks I'm weird because I act like I'm immune to the pressures to eat many of the foods we've talked about in this chapter. How can it be that some people are drawn to these foods while others don't seem to be influenced by them at all? Either they have refined the ability to resist the urges, or they simply don't have the urges.

Resembling Addiction

Rats also like salt, sugar and fat. To answer the questions about differences in our urges for these foods scientists did a study with rats. It's well known that rats (and humans) will do a certain amount of work or effort to get a reward. When rats were given a taste of slightly sweetened drops versus plain water, they preferred the sweetened drops and will work to get it. To get another taste of the sweetened drops, the rats had to press a little lever.[4] Some rats pushed the lever up to 10 times to get the sweetened drops, while others pushed just a few times and gave up. For them, the work wasn't worth the effort to get the sweet drops—kind of like me and a cinnamon roll. I like the flavor, but not enough to buy one and certainly not enough to make an entire batch from scratch. I just don't care enough. Other rats, however, really like the taste and will work very hard to repeat the experience. What's the difference between the two groups of rats? Both were given a taste of the solution and both had to do the same amount of work to get the drops again. The difference it seems is in how much pleasure the rats experience from tasting the drops. If the pleasure was intense, they worked harder to get it. If the pleasure sensation was so-so, they really didn't have a lot to gain by all the hard work. Some have suggested that the difference lies in how much our brains respond to the initial taste. It appears that some people have more of the receptors and brain chemicals that respond to sweet, sugar and fat. The difference may be due to genetic differences in how the taste is perceived, felt and recorded. In a sense, Cinnabon's business model may actually act just like a genetic test. The fresh smell and taste of their cinnamon rolls may have a greater impact on certain, genetically prone individuals. I find that I can walk by a fresh cinnamon roll and think nothing of it, while others may be impulsively drawn to it because of the differences in how we perceive the cinnamon roll eating experience.

As I visit with people about this I find that women seem to struggle with the taste, crave, repeat cycle more so than men. There isn't any survey data to back this up, but anecdotally, women may be more prone to food addiction. They often tell me of intense cravings for foods high in salt, sugar and fat. This doesn't mean that men don't suffer from the same addictions, they do, but perhaps the prevalence of food addiction is higher for women than for men. As to why, I can only guess.

We can learn even more from the rats. As the concentration of sugar in the drops increased from 0 to 10% and higher, the amount of work the rats were willing to exert increased. But once the concentration reached 30%, the rats were unwilling to put out the same amount of work. The highest concentrations crossed the "too much sugar doesn't taste as good limit." Have you ever had a glass of lemonade that was too sweet? You probably made a funny face and quickly put the glass down. We learn two things from these rats. Just like us, they prefer sugared drinks over non-sugared drinks and will work to get the extra sugar. But there is a limit as to how much sugar is enough. Something about the taste of sugar changes the rats' preferences. The pleasure they get from the sweet taste makes them want to come back for more, even if there is a price to be paid for the opportunity. From this research, we can also learn that if rats had money, they'd make great customers.

Just like sweetened drops, rats responded the same way to drops that contain fat. With each increased concentration, the rats were willing to do more work, until it reached a certain point where the reward was not worth the effort.[5] When drops contained sugar and fat, the amount of work the rats were willing to do was even greater than work done for sugar or fat drops alone. The combination of the two flavors made them crave the opportunity even more and they were willing to work significantly harder to repeat it. Remember, a craving occurs when our brains tell us how badly we want to repeat a previously enjoyable experience. Researchers have also studied the addictive nature of drugs on rats. They found that there was absolutely no difference between the amount of work rats will do for sugar, salt and fat and the amount of work they are willing to do to get another hit of cocaine. Rats will work just as hard to get more sugar and fat as they will to get cocaine.[6]

This brings us back to the question of whether or not foods can be addictive. Consider this email I received:

Dear Dr. Aldana:

I've struggled with addiction for years. It is a constant battle to control my thoughts because every day, throughout the day, I think of getting some more. Regardless of how it affects my marriage, my work or my health, I still seek it out and once I start, it's extremely hard to stop. I feel terrible about myself because I know I shouldn't do it, but after a while my feelings of depression get replaced with cravings to do it again and once I start, there is no stopping me. I have a complete loss of control while I'm doing it. Most times I can't even remember how much I've taken. I'm really good at hiding it from others. My family has no idea I'm struggling. I wish I could stop, but it's really hard. Every time I'm successful at stopping, time passes and eventually I let my guard down and do it again. It's like I'm trapped in the vicious cycle. What can I do?

From this letter it's not easy to determine what issue this person was struggling with. He could be struggling with drug addiction, alcohol abuse or even sex addiction. One thing is for sure, it sounds like he has all the classic symptoms of an addiction. He thinks about it often, he keeps doing it despite the fact that it is destroying his relationships and health. He cycles through use, remorse, depression, and reuse and feels almost powerless to stop. This letter is from my friend Paul who I introduced in an earlier chapter. Paul's addiction is with delicious tasting foods. His consumption, remorse, and depression and re-consumption are based on eating his favorite salt, sugar and fat-laced foods. He is an individual who can open a carton of ice cream and not stop until the entire container has been emptied. He's the frequent traveler Cinnabon loves. Eventually, he may be the obese, diabetic patient at the nursing home who has had a leg amputated and will die 16 years before his time—all because he is trapped in the food addiction cycle.

To me, this description sounds just like an addiction story that could be about anyone addicted to drugs or alcohol. I'm not the only one who sees the similarities between the cycle of addiction from drugs and the cycle of addiction from food. Most scientists aren't quite ready to declare that food addiction is real. They prefer to call it the addiction hypothesis.[7] In order for something to be officially labeled as addictive it must have research unequivocally demonstrating that certain foods can cause the classic symptoms of addiction. Under this process, it is only a matter of time before psychologists start making a clinically accepted diagnosis of food addiction. And when it happens, a huge number of Americans will finally have confirmation for what they've always known: it's really hard not to eat processed, delicious tasting foods.

We're all trapped in this vicious cycle. We have a prehistoric preference for foods with salt, sugar and fat. We buy them, taste them, crave them, and then we do it all over again. The food industry responds with more and more foods that contain varying amounts of these flavors and suddenly we are surrounded by a food culture that encourages too much of the wrong kinds of foods. The quantity and quality of our food has changed. The outcome of this cycle is increased body weight and more chronic diseases. The salt we crave causes high blood pressure. The processed and sugary foods we desire cause a spike in blood glucose which can lead to diabetes. The fats we consume are the building materials our bodies need to make cholesterol. When we eat these addictive foods, our blood fats are altered and we eventually develop cardiovascular disease.

What Difference Does It Make?

Does it really matter what we call our relationship with food? Probably not, because regardless of the name we apply to the overconsumption of unhealthy foods, the outcome is the same. If we continue to consume a diet that is characterized by large amounts of salt, sugar and fat our prehistoric body will eventually stop functioning normally, chronic diseases will ensue and we'll suffer a premature, painful death.

The manipulation of our diet by food producers is our own fault. Originally, these engineered foods were not thrust upon us by a food industry bent on world domination. No, our highly palatable foods choices were influenced by you and I every time we purchased indulgent foods carefully created with salt, sugar and fat. As our preferences for these flavors became known, the food industry responded with more of the same. The more of them we eat, the more money they make and the more time and effort they put into creating even more delicious foods. Without exception, every fast food company in America has created new menu items that exploit this flavor profile.

Our desire for foods that fulfill our salt, sugar and fat cravings have now become so common that it has dramatically altered the total amount of food consumed in the U.S. In 1970, the average American consumed 2,300 mg of sodium every day.[8] Today, our sodium intake is much higher at 3,500 mg—an increase of 1,100 mg per day.[9] To put this into perspective, 1,100 mg of sodium is the same amount of sodium found in seven pieces of bread or 29 cans of Pepsi or four small Wendy's fries or three Taco Bell tacos. Almost all of the sodium we eat today comes from processed foods and fast foods. The added salt from your salt shaker is irrelevant compared to the total amount of salt found in the foods we purchase. This is important because about one-third of the U.S. population has high blood pressure; a leading cause of cardiovascular disease.

If all you do is lower the amount of sodium you eat, you can lower your blood pressure by as much as 11mm. That's enough to save tens of thousands of lives each year, and that amount of improvement is more than you can get from medication.[10] Reducing your consumption of sodium is easier said than done because most of the processed and fast foods you purchase are loaded with sodium. If you purchase food, and we all do, it's extremely difficult to avoid eating lots of sodium. The food industry wants to sell lots of food, and they know that extra sodium makes you crave and buy more. Expecting the food industry to voluntarily use less sodium in their foods is like asking the oil industry to charge less for gasoline because the high prices might cause drivers undue financial stress. As we'll see later, the whole notion of asking the food industry to self-regulate by providing safer, healthier foods is misguided and ineffective.

In Chapter 1, I showed a chart that documents our increased consumption of sugars and fat. Here is the chart again. Now that we've talked about how our desires for flavorful foods have altered the U.S. food landscape the chart takes on new meaning. Since the discovery that humans really like salt, sugar and fat, the total amount of production and consumption of these three ingredients has risen dramatically.

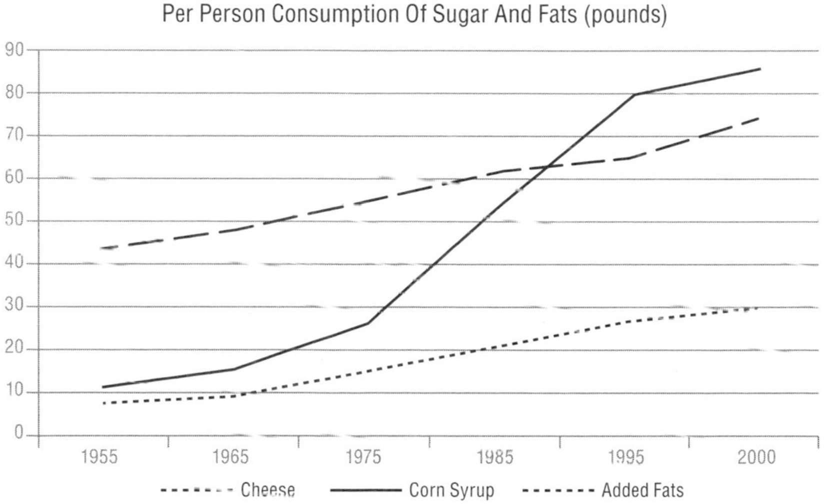

http://www.usda.gov/factbook/chapter2.pdf

Just like salt, our consumption of fats and sugars has increased and will continue to increase dramatically. There is little that can be done to stop this trend. People like you and I really like the taste of foods that have these ingredients and we're willing to buy more.

When you think about how to improve your health it is important to know what you are up against. You are up against a massive infrastructure that can quickly and efficiently produce the fat, sugar and salt-infused foods you and almost every other American loves so much. Farmers grow massive amounts of soybeans, canola and corn to supply the ever-increasing demand. Every aspect of our current food supply, from farmer's fields to the dinner table has been altered to support our demand for these flavorful foods. Hundreds of thousands of workers are required to create and deliver these foods to the masses. A good portion of our economy is based on the growth, processing and selling of massive quantities of food—food that results in the development of chronic diseases and are directly responsible for the obesity and diabetes epidemics that surround us. Worst of all, there is an even bigger element of this new food economy and culture: greed. Large sums of money are being made by the current system. If you trace the dollars you spend on food back through the food chain, you'll see that each player in the system profits from your purchase. Some more than others, but overall, your money drives the entire system. If your good health requires others to make less money, the money makers in the system will almost always win.

There are two sides to your battle for better health. You, the consumer, and your desire for a long, healthy life are on one side. Fighting against you is the U.S. food industrial complex with all of its financial and political fire power. This is a David vs. Goliath battle and you and your desires for good health are getting your butt kicked. Unless you understand your enemy and are able to use all the right tools and weapons, you don't stand a chance of winning.

There are only two ways you are going to win this battle. The first is for you to wait for reinforcements. State and federal governments and health professionals will need to convince the food industry to stop selling unhealthy foods. Many concerned people are working hard to make this happen and I applaud their efforts. Unfortunately, experience shows that this approach is futile, and even if they do succeed, their efforts will be too little too late. This approach is well-intended, but ultimately pointless because it's unrealistic to expect corporations and industries to pursue public health more aggressively than quarterly profits. I'm afraid the cavalry is not coming to the rescue.

The second way to survive this fight is to drop your weapon and run. Undoubtedly, this is not the bravest strategy, but it is a survival strategy. Leave the battle as fast as you can. Within your homes and places of work you can create and live in a new culture of health within our unhealthy culture. Isolate yourself, your family, coworkers or neighbors from the unhealthy cultural influences that surround you. Once you've retreated, build a moat that keeps the unhealthy aspects of our culture at bay. My wife builds a moat around our home when she tells our kids and I, "Don't bring that (delicious food) into the house, it's contraband." These somewhat different living arrangements are not intended to become a post-apocalyptic survival compound, but a simple real world attempt to "live in the world, but not be completely of the world." We still live in our homes and have all the conveniences of our modern age, but we can select which parts of our culture we wish to participate in. Carefully avoiding the unhealthy influences is the only realistic long-term solution to achieving and maintaining good health.

Don't get too worried about the food addictions we all seem to have. Once you have your new culture created, you'll learn effective strategies to not only avoid the addiction in the first place, but how to break the buy, taste, crave and repeat cycle.

Island Native

My name is Max Bradshaw. I am retired and I live in Columbus, Ohio. For most of my life I have lived an unhealthy lifestyle. I ate, drank and was merry, but after years of putting my lifestyle second, I had a heart attack. Following my heart attack my lifestyle still didn't change and I had a stroke. After two life-threatening events the only thing that got me to change was realizing my kids and grandkids needed me.

Admitting I needed to change was hard and when I did change the first thing to go was my smoking. I smoked in my twenties and quit, but started again 20 years later. What really helped me quit was a painful knee surgery that helped me focus on pain rather than the need for a smoke. I used medication that helped reduce my cravings. For me, changing my diet was very hard because my life was built around food. At work I was given doughnuts, soda-pop, full spread breakfasts and large meals because that is how my work rewarded me for working hard. When I decided to change I had to ask myself at meals, "Do I really need that much?" I realized that the portions I was eating were huge and I only needed a fourth of what I was eating. Sharing meals with my wife was one of the easiest ways for me to reduce my portions. We order and cook all our meals so that each of us has enough to enjoy our meal without getting stuffed.

Although changing my diet has been very important to me I have also committed myself to exercising. Every morning I begin my day with exercise. I work out on an elliptical and treadmill, and if the weather is good I head outside. All of my change wouldn't have been possible without such a supportive wife. She has cooked healthy meals for me and has taken extra special care of me. I also want to keep doing this because my grandkids need a grandpa who they can look up to. In some sort of way I also want to defy my dad's expectations one last time by living longer than he did, which was 85. The only way I can do that is if I stick to my changes. I would tell others, "Nobody will do this for you. If you can't do it yourself be ready to expect the consequences."

CHAPTER 5

We Have Changed

ASK YOURSELF THIS QUESTION: WHO REALLY CARES ABOUT YOUR HEALTH? THE MOST OBVIOUS ANSWER IS YOU. NO ONE HAS MORE TO GAIN OR LOSE THAN YOU DO, SO NATURALLY YOU'RE AT THE TOP OF THE LIST. Unless you've been a complete jerk, your close family members and friends also want you to have a long, healthy life. They care about your health. What about your employer? Does your employer care about your health? Most employers care because a healthy employee is a productive and happy employee. Occasionally, some employers treat their employees like family; they are sincerely interested and concerned about their employees and their families. However, once we leave the influences of close family, friends and some employers, honest, heart-felt interest in your health starts to weaken.

Let's ask this question a different way. Who stands to lose money if we improve our lifestyles and work hard at trying to have good health? If all Americans started adopting healthy behaviors, one of the first businesses to suffer the consequences would be the tobacco industry. Smoke shops around the country would close, many tobacco manufacturing jobs would be lost, tobacco farmers would go out of business and stock holders would see the value of their tobacco investments decline. The U.S. economy as a whole would take a hit, but not too badly because most tobacco companies in the U.S. also sell a lot of tobacco to other countries. A healthier U.S. population would impact the tobacco industry, but they'd survive because they've reduced their risk by selling their deadly product into a global market.

What about the food industry? If we all started eating less salt, sugar and fat, who would lose money? Every person and company that is involved with making and selling foods with these ingredients would make less money. The beverage industry, farmers, fast food companies, food corporations, advertising companies, dairy farmers, grocery stores, restaurants and specialty food companies would see fewer sales. No doubt, many people would lose their jobs. Obviously we have to eat something, so additional jobs would be needed to make healthier foods, but the financial losses in some food markets would be staggering. What about hospitals and health care providers? Unlike every other country in the world, health care in the U.S. is big business. Health care providers exist to make profits and provide health care. They make money treating disease. If there is less disease to treat, there is less money to make. Drug manufacturers, medical equipment manufacturers, health care lawyers and insurance companies will all lose money if Americans had better health. Kidney dialysis centers are big business and 91% of patients in those centers are there because of poor lifestyles and diabetes. A healthy population would reduce their patient supply by 91%. Every month, most of us pay health insurance premiums to insurance companies who use our money to process health claims, pay for medical services and to make a profit. If we were all healthy, fewer medical services would be needed, fewer claims would be processed and insurance companies would make less money. Stock holders would see the value of these companies go down. A really healthy population is bad for profits if you are in the disease treatment business. How about pharmaceutical companies? If we are all healthy, the need for medications would plunge. Good health is bad for businesses if you are in the business of making money on treating poor health. I'm not suggesting that all of these industries don't care about your health—they do, but they also care more about making money.

What does all this really have to do with you and your health? As we talk about trying to live a longer, healthier life you will be more likely to succeed if you understand the forces working for and against you. How many people do you know who have actually lost weight and were able to keep it off? Most likely not very many because the forces that push people to gain weight are greater than the forces working to help people maintain a healthy weight. In a sense, we are all influenced by those who stand to make money from the current culture and though they may not admit it openly, industries that profit from our culture are actively working against you and your efforts to be healthy. Behind all the pleasantries and public good will, we are surrounded by companies, industries and even our own government that are way more interested in maintaining the status quo and making money than helping you and I get healthy. This conflict is at the core of our struggle for better health.

Two Sides To Our Health Battles

Let's start with an extreme example of how this works. About 21% of Americans smoke. This percentage of Americans will die about 14 years before the average person who doesn't smoke.[1] One in every five deaths in the U.S. is caused by tobacco, and worldwide tobacco causes five million deaths every year.[2] In short, tobacco users die way before their time and during their lives they suffer painful cancers and diseases that cost all of us an enormous amount of money to treat. The taxes and insurance premiums non-smokers pay help support the $198 billion we spend each year to treat smoking-related illnesses. With such a horrible impact on life, health and society how is it even conceivable that we don't do even more to discourage tobacco use? Here is where those "forces" I've been referring to kick in.

What would happen if all of the 65 million American smokers decided to quit? All those smokers would instantly have an extra $2,000 to $5,000 per year to spend on anything except tobacco. The average cost of a package of cigarettes is $5.58 per pack, or about 30 cents per cigarette. Tobacco farmers would be out of work. Some tobacco companies, hospitals, doctors and drug manufacturers would go bankrupt or experience dramatic downsizing. Funeral homes and ambulance services would lose substantial business. Many of those whose lives have been disrupted by the change would cry out to their state, local and federal governments for help. Tobacco lobbyists would start hounding congress for direct financial support for legislation to support American jobs.

When it comes to government, some states have different approaches to tobacco use. The state of New York is tired of paying for the additional health care costs of smokers, so they raised the cost of a pack of cigarettes to $9.11. Not wanting to hurt farmers, doctors, hospitals, advertising companies or the tobacco industries, states like Virginia and Missouri keep the price down to $3.90 a pack. They don't want to hurt local economies by imposing government mandated taxes on tobacco. In states like Virginia and Missouri they are content having non-smokers subsidize the extra societal costs incurred by tobacco users. Of the 10 states with the lowest taxes on tobacco, most are tobacco-producing states. Their state politicians are more interested in protecting the tobacco industry than their citizens' health. Of course, the higher cost of cigarettes has a direct impact on reducing the amount people smoke. Every 10% increase in the cost of cigarettes reduces smoking by three to five percent and it reduces the number of young adults and kids who smoke by three to seven percent.[3] Raising the taxes on tobacco ultimately keeps people from starting and it reduces the amount people smoke. In short, it saves lives and saves money. Unfortunately, despite these efforts millions of Americans continue to smoke and a solid 21% of the U.S. population consists of tobacco users. This is a perfect example of the battles that exist between you and your desires for good health and all the organizations, companies and politicians who care more about making money and supporting the status quo than the quality of your life. It's the conflict that arises when society supports values that contradict each other. Tobacco kills prematurely and costs society billions of dollars each year, and yet state and federal governments continue to allow the tobacco industry to advertise, sell and heavily market their product.

In precisely the same manner, you and I value good health and try to exercise regularly and have a healthy diet while many industries and politicians have a different set of values. They value the economy, profits, jobs and maintaining the status quo. So it makes perfect sense that these stakeholders will do practically anything to defend that status quo. For example, when efforts have been made to reduce the amount of sodium in our food, the food industry is quick to react. The president of the Salt Institute, Richard Hanneman, has come out publicly and forcefully against anything that encourages people to eat less salt. Like the tobacco industry, the attack is not about health, it's about maintaining profitable businesses and to make this attack successful, they twist the argument away from the scientific evidence that links sodium consumption to poor health and make it a moral issue. People get angry and emotional about moral issues. Hence, the Salt Institute says, "We don't think it's possible for the government to legislate or regulate a reduction in sodium content. It would be like legislating morality." This takes the issue of adding salt to your food so you'll buy more and turns it into a heated argument about government interfering in your morality. It takes the profitable practice of adding salt to food and hides it behind the sacred protection of your God-given rights to believe and live as you choose. According to those in the salt industry, it would be immoral NOT to allow the food industry to add as much salt as they want to the foods you consume. When industry starts making protection of the status quo a moral issue, they are really saying that any attempt to interfere would be immoral. And as any blue-blooded American knows, if you are immoral you will go to hell. I hear hell is supposed to be a bad place, so unless you want to go to hell, don't mess with the salt industry…and we don't.

The Salt Institute is a North American trade organization charged with the protection and promotion of the salt industry. Between 1983 and 1998 salt purchases have increased by 86% and salt sales have increased by 55%.[4] At exactly the same time, the consumption of sugar-sweetened beverages (think soda) increased by 135%. A higher level of dietary sodium results in a greater degree of thirst, especially for carbonated drinks.[5] If these two trends are related, and it appears that they are, it is likely that the added salt and the added calories from sweetened beverages are contributing directly to our obesity epidemic. The salt industry is making more money than ever on consumers who crave high-sodium foods and beverages.

Obviously the salt industry is not the tobacco industry, but the conflict between the values of the salt industry and your desires for better health is the same conflict we have with cigarette manufacturers. The salt industry wants to maintain a steady stream of profits even if that means you live with chronic disease and die a premature death.

So we're stuck. Foods full of salt, sugar and fat are delicious, inexpensive and integrated into the very fabric of our culture. Because we like the taste of these foods so much, we buy more and more and the food industry is only meeting the additional demand. We created the demand, they supply the products; any attempt to alter the supply of unhealthy foods by raising taxes or adding new regulations will be skewed as immoral by anyone who stands to lose money with the changes. Once this process begins, there is almost no way to stop it. Our entire U.S. food culture is impacted by this seemingly unstoppable cycle. But we don't think about these cycles, we go about our daily lives almost oblivious to what the salt industry is doing or what the food industry is saying. We only stop to wonder what's going on when our health is negatively impacted or when we gain weight. This is one reason children and young adults don't typically care about any of this. Despite their unhealthy behaviors, they can ride the crest of youth, maintaining what appears to be good health. They may gain a little weight, but they feel just fine living the way they do. Indeed, you can seemingly eat garbage for 40 years and still not feel the pains and aches of mortality. Of course, good health after age 40 has to be earned with years of healthy living.

Inside The Aldana Home

I have children who attend public schools here in my hometown. Each school in my area has numerous vending machines that sell candies, chips and soda. They are available and open to student purchases all day. These vending machines are there for a very specific purpose: to make money. One school district in my area makes $3 million a year from Pepsi sales alone. The beverage companies and the school districts make lots of money when the kids spend their spare money on candy and soda.

Many states are trying to pass laws that would restrict the sale of unhealthy foods in public schools. As soon as the committees start to consider these laws, the lobbyists from the food industry go on the attack. They spend money countering any effort to remove unhealthy food. They donate money to state legislators and in some states they out number poorly funded health advocates by 10 to 1. This money helps legislators get re-elected and as a return favor for the generous donations, these bills rarely get put to a vote. Food lobbyists and even some school administrators fight these bills at every turn. This has been going on in Washington, California, Pennsylvania and many other states including my own state of Colorado. Health teachers in our schools teach about good health and good nutrition while at the exact same time the schools themselves are making millions off of junk food sales. All U.S. states allow public schools to profit from exactly the same foods we're teaching our children not to eat.

This occurs mostly in junior high and high schools where older kids have more expendable income and have the ability to purchase the food themselves. Most elementary schools draw a line and think that selling junk food to small children is inappropriate, bordering on exploitation, but as soon as they get a little older and have a little more spending money, vending machines appear…let the exploitation begin! Few changes are being made because the schools and food vendors are unwilling to compromise this source of money. While schools make money, the health of our children is ignored. The problems associated with trying to serve two masters has a direct, daily impact on the health of our children.

How We've Changed

In the past 30 years Americans have added an additional 570 calories to their daily food intake. Our specific eating habits have changed so that on average we now eat 570 more calories every day. What has so drastically changed and is the food industry responsible for getting us into this mess? And if we can identify these changes is it possible to reverse them?

In my opinion these are some of the most important questions we can ask if we are serious about improving our health. Scientists have been asking these exact questions and have found some very important findings. Unfortunately, the public rarely learns about them.

Researchers have been doing national nutrition surveys for decades. Every five or 10 years they do another national survey. The data collected is analyzed and a picture of long-term changes in our nutrition is revealed. It is from these data sets that we discovered we are eating 570 more calories every day compared to 30 years ago.[6] Although increases in total calories tells us the results, they don't tell us how it happened. It's clear that we eat more calories now than in the past, but what are we doing differently that is responsible for the added calories and how has the self-serving food industry contributed to these changes? I think you may be surprised at what we have learned.

It's Not Only How Much We Eat, it's also How Often We Eat

How many times do you eat in a day? Consider these four typical eating times in your answer: breakfast, lunch, dinner and snacking times. If you are a straight breakfast, lunch and dinner kind of person, the answer is three. In 1977, the average number of eating times for most Americans was 3.8.[6] Remember, this is an average of thousands of people. Many reported three, some reported five, others said they ate four times per day; when all the individual reports were averaged it came to 3.8 eating periods each day. Today, the average number of times we eat is 4.9. Somehow in the last 30 years we have added 1.1 extra eating times to our day. Most likely, people aren't reporting that they ate two breakfasts or three dinners. Most likely, individuals report eating three meals per day, with the extra eating times being snacking. Sure enough, when we look at the data closer most of the extra eating periods consist of snacking. Buying a big cup of soda at the gas station or grabbing a bag of chips from the vending machine counts as one of these extra eating times.

So what has changed that makes us eat more often? In the past 30 years we've increased the number of hours we work. Recently, 86% of males and 66% of females reported working more than 40 hours per week. More time at work means less time to cook and fewer meals eaten at home. I tell my children that not long ago there was a time when gas stations only sold gas. You might find soda, but rarely any food. We used to call them gas stations, but now we just call them convenience stores that happen to also sell gas. Many of us get some of our meals at convenience stores. If we don't stop to get some food, we stop to get some coffee. On a recent trip to Nebraska, I was working with one of the managers of a construction company. We spent several days visiting worksites across several states. I was surprised to see that every day between 1:00 and 4:00 p.m. he would drive miles out of our way to find a Starbucks where he would purchase two large cups of fat and sugar infused coffee. If you counted his breakfast, lunch and dinner, his eating events always averaged at least four per day. And most of those events occurred with him eating food outside of his home.

Food eaten outside the home can be either a regular meal or a snack. The Starbucks visits were in the snack category. Perhaps we eat more times during the day because we are home less often, working, traveling and playing in areas where fast food choices are plentiful and convenient. One of the best reasons we eat more times per day is because it has become so easy to do so. Americans are cooking meals at home much less often than they used to. Why cook, when you can buy food already cooked or food that is extremely easy to prepare? Even though preparing food at home is cheaper and healthier, Americans are willing to spend more on food that is convenient and precooked.

Percentage Of Your Money Used To Buy Food Outside The Home[7]

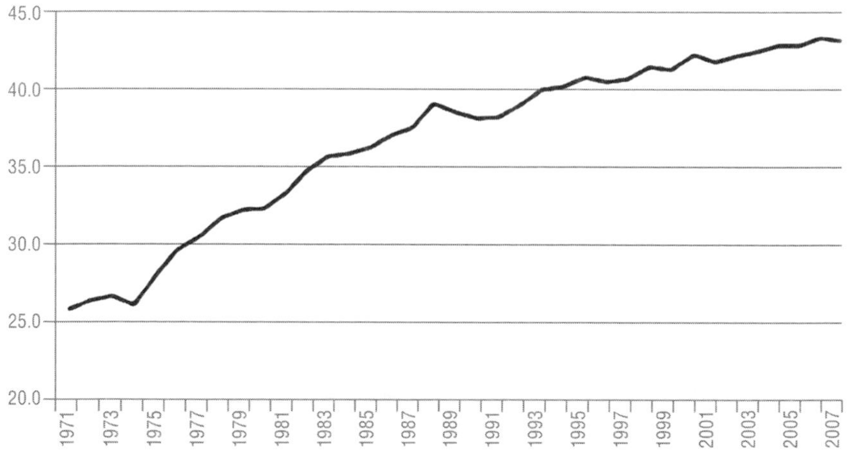

In 1900, two percent of all meals were eaten outside the home. Today, 50% of all meals are eaten away from home. We're also spending more money on food outside the home, almost double what it was 40 years ago. Food is one of those monthly expenditures we all budget for. The amount we spend on food has increased and each year more of our hard-earned dollars are being spent on food purchased and eaten outside the home.

There are several reasons why this trend will continue. For one, there are more women employed outside the home, which often means two-earner households and higher incomes. At the same time, there are more affordable and convenient fast food outlets, increased advertising and promotion by large restaurant chains and smaller families (which means fewer mouths to feed). Individually, each of these changes in our demographics makes it easier and more convenient to eat out and to eat more often.

Not So Healthy Away From Home

Maybe you are wondering why we should even care about whether or not we eat food that has been prepared outside or inside the home. However, it's extremely important because the weight gain and chronic diseases America is experiencing are directly related to the quantity and quality of food we eat. The foods we consume at home are generally healthier than the foods we consume outside the home.

Every meal eaten outside the home has 134 more calories than a meal eaten at home. One meal a week eaten outside the home translates to an extra two pounds of body fat every year.

On a national basis, every meal eaten outside the home per week translates to two extra pounds of body fat per year.[8] Those convenient, delicious, inexpensive meals eaten outside the home contain about 134 more calories than meals eaten in the home. If what we said about salt, sugar and fat are true and they really are the preferred ingredients for restaurants and fast foods, then meals eaten outside the home should have higher amounts of these ingredients. This is exactly what the USDA found when they compared the nutrition content of meals eaten at home and meals eaten outside the home. Compared to meals eaten at home, fast food and restaurant food has 22% fewer fruit servings, 30% fewer vegetables and 20% fewer whole grains.[8] As expected, these foods also have six percent more fat (mostly saturated fat) and significantly more sugar.[9] Those extra 134 calories in meals eaten outside the home come from added fat, sugar and fewer fruits, vegetables and whole grains. These changes increase the calories in the foods you eat and make them more energy dense.

Compared To Meals Eaten At Home, Meals Eaten Outside The Home Have Fewer Fruits, Vegetables, And Whole Grains And Have More Fat And Sugar

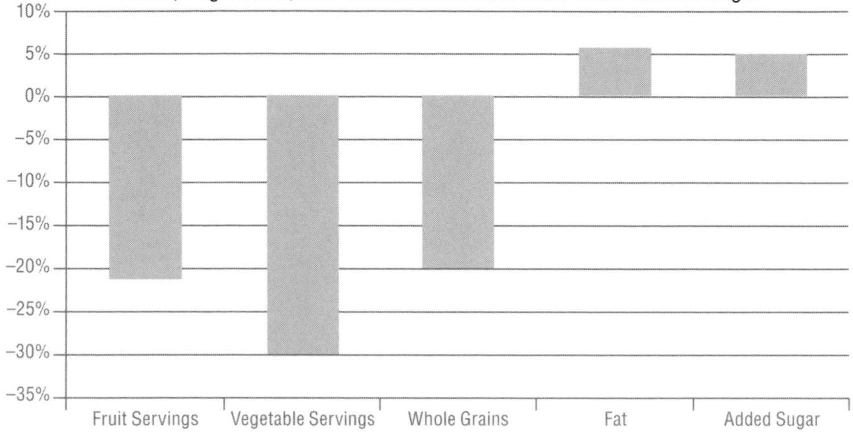

If you take children to eat meals outside the home they too will get more calories than if they were eating meals at home. From 1977 to 2006 children increased daily calorie consumption by 180 calories and all of this increase was caused by consuming higher density foods outside the home.[10] The increased calorie content of foods eaten outside the home is believed to be one of the leading causes of childhood obesity.

To be sure, there is one variable that predicts obesity better than most. It's even a better predictor than exercise, education level or income. It's the number of times a person eats outside the home.[11] The frequency of eating foods from restaurants serving fried chicken, burgers, pizza, fried fish and other convenience foods is directly associated with excessive body fat. That's because these foods have a higher energy density. They have higher amounts of total fat and saturated fat and lower levels of fiber.

More Calories Than Ever

The ingredients of foods eaten outside the home include more salt, sugar and fat, which means they have a higher energy density. Again, energy density is a measure of how many calories there are per ounce. For example, a half-pound of fruit or vegetables has about 54 calories. But, if you eat a half-pound of typical snack food like cookies, cake, pie, ice cream or chocolate you are eating about 20 times more calories. A half cup of chocolate has 1,100 calories.[12] This means that your snack foods can have almost 20 times the calories for the same amount of food. A half-pound of your favorite potato chips can have 1,300 calories. And even if you eat the "reduced fat" version you are still getting 1,120 calories. Foods and snacks eaten outside the home have more calories because they have more salt, fat and sugar.

Compared to our ancient ancestors, our diet today is much more calorie dense, which means that our food has more energy per ounce than in any other time in human history. Since our food is more energy dense, the next logical question is: What, if any, impact does this have on our health? Maybe when we eat foods high in calories our appetites adjust and we eat less. Maybe we keep eating the same amount of food and just keep consuming more calories.

Scientists at Harvard University got 50,000 middle-aged women to document what they were eating for several weeks.[13] With that information, they calculated the energy density of their diets, and they also measured their health and health risks. Then they stopped studying the women for eight years. After eight years, they relocated most of the women and once again measured their health risks. They discovered that those women who had the highest energy density also had gained the most weight. They were also able to show that women who had high density diets ate more total fat, saturated fat and trans fat, and they also ate fewer fruits and vegetables. The higher the energy density of the foods they ate, the more weight they gained. This shows a direct relationship between the energy density of our diet and weight gain. The more high fat, high sugar, low fruit, low vegetable foods we consume, the more we weigh.

At the same time, researchers at Penn State University did a similar study.[14] They measured the body weight and energy density of a group of women then followed them for six years. It didn't matter how much they weighed in the beginning. If their diet included lots of energy dense foods, they gained weight. The ones who gained the most weight were women who ate baked desserts, refined grains, few fruits, vegetables and cereal. Women with low energy density diets were the only ones who didn't gain weight over the six years. The researchers also showed that those who ate lower energy density diets ate more meals at the table and fewer meals in front of the television. Maybe it's not the act of watching television that makes us fat, but rather the energy density of the foods we eat while watching television that is to blame.

Most of us don't talk about food with technical terms like "energy density" or "eating opportunities per day." We talk about food taste, cost and convenience. We talk about foods according to whether we think our children will or won't eat them. Take oatmeal for example. My family and I eat a lot of oatmeal. I buy it in a 50-pound bag that lasts us a year or two. It's easy to cook, tastes good and gets even better when you add fruit and nuts. My bowl of oatmeal contains oatmeal, some fruit, nuts and a pinch of brown sugar—about 150 calories.

However, the food industry doesn't make much money on a boring 50 pound bag of oatmeal. So, rather than selling plain oatmeal they sell Quaker Dinosaur Eggs Brown Sugar Oatmeal. It has 200 calories per serving and has the following ingredients:

Whole Grain Rolled Oats (With Oat Bran), Sugar, Dinosaur Egg Shaped Pieces (Sugar, Dextrose, Partially Hydrogenated Soybean and/or Cottonseed Oil, Maltodextrin, Confectioner's Glaze, Magnesium Stearate, Soy Lecithin (An Emulsifier), Modified Corn Starch, Red 40 Lake, Yellow 6 Lake, Yellow 5 Lake, Artificial Color, Blue 1 Lake , Bleached Beeswax. Carnauba Wax, Natural and Artificial Flavors), Natural and Artificial Flavors. Bone Shaped Pieces (Sugar, Rice Flour, Confectioner's Glaze, Partially Hydrogenated Cottonseed and Soybean Oil, Cornstarch, Dextrin, Modified Food Starch, Cellulose Gum, Carnauba Wax, Carrageenan, Bleached Beeswax, Artificial Color, Gum Tragacanth, Yellow 5, Artificial Flavor), Natural and Artificial Flavors (Contains Wheat, Soy, and Milk Components), Salt, Calcium Carbonate (A Source of Calcium), Guar Gum, Caramel Color, Niacinamide (One of the B Vitamins), Vitamin A Palmitate, Reduced Iron, Pyridoxine Hydrochloride (One of the B Vitamins), Riboflavin (One of the B Vitamins), Thiamin Mononitrate (One of the B Vitamins), Folic Acid (One of the B Vitamins)

Long ingredient list made short—this oatmeal has been processed until it is unrecognizable. Besides the added sugars, artificial colors and other ingredients, kids will still love it because it has a cool name and it's full of dinosaur egg and bone-shaped candy. What kid wouldn't like candy for breakfast?

This is just one of hundreds of thousands of food products that have been altered and turned into a high energy density food. It's a money maker for the food industry. The horrific list of ingredients and amount of processing required to make this food are reason enough to avoid it, but we still purchase foods like this because we trust food manufacturers and we respond to effective food marketing. We're convinced that any food with oatmeal and vitamins and minerals must be good for us, so we buy and consume. The downside of all this is that we now know that high energy dense foods, like this oatmeal, are directly related to weight gain and we're gaining this weight faster than ever.

The amount of calories we now eat has gone up, but there is also a big increase in the number of calories we drink. Drinking a sugared drink with a meal greatly increases the meal's energy density. If you eat a meal and drink water, you typically eat until you are full. If you eat the same meal with a sugared beverage, you eat the same amount of food, but you get all the extra calories from the beverage. When we drink calorie-packed sugary drinks our bodies don't tell us to eat less. We treat the sugary beverage just like we treat water, we use it to quench our thirst, not to satisfy our hunger.[15] Calories in our drinks often don't get counted mentally, but they do get counted on the weight scale.

In children, obesity is 1.6 times more likely with each serving of sugar-sweetened drinks consumed per day.[16] The more sugared drinks a child consumes, the more likely he or she is to be obese. You can even predict how much body fat a child will have by measuring how much sugared drinks they consume per day. What about milk shakes? Even though we sometimes think of these as beverages, they really aren't. They are more like partially melted ice cream. When we consume a malt or a milk shake, or even slightly melted ice cream, our stomachs recognize these as solid foods. These foods are cold and filling. There's no fooling the stomach into thinking we haven't consumed anything, we feel full quicker and we stop eating sooner. Just because these calories do get detected, I'm not giving you permission to eat all the ice cream and milk shakes you want. That would be taking these research findings a bit too far and would be detrimental to your long-term health.

If you think about this for a minute, it all makes sense. Our bodies are ancient, adapted to live and thrive in an environment drastically different than the one we live in today. For 100,000 years, the only beverage with any calories was mother's milk and after infancy we stopped drinking it. Because the only beverage available to humans was water, our bodies have become accustomed to calorie-free water to quench thirst. Today, we still drink lots of water, it's just mixed with carbonation, sugar, high-fructose corn syrup or alcohol and the calories in these drinks are in addition to our normal food consumption.

Portion Distortion

Our memories fade with time. Can you remember what a typical food serving looked like 10, 20 or 30 years ago? You may have the suspicious feeling that the amount of food in a single serving has gone up. But how much? Our memory has changed and we have forgotten what a normal serving size looks like. Even though we've forgotten what food sizes were in the past, we still sense the increase when we get served a meal and marvel at how much food has been heaped on to the plate. Let's see just how familiar you are with how much our food servings have changed. Here are five typical foods: salty snacks, soft drinks, hamburgers, French fries and Mexican food. In the late 1970s national surveys were conducted on these foods to determine how many calories were in a single serving of each. Twenty years later they conducted the same survey and measured the caloric content of a serving of the same foods. The serving sizes for all five increased substantially. Compared to the late 1970s, the salty snacks we have today have 93 more calories per serving, soft drinks 49 more calories, hamburgers 97 more calories, French fries 58 more calories and Mexican food a whopping 133 more calories.[17] The last time I had Mexican food, my meal was not served on a plate. It was served on an 18-inch platter and had enough food for two or three people. We have forgotten what servings sizes were historically and now we suffer from portion distortion—perceiving large portion sizes as appropriate amounts to eat at a single eating occasion.[18] Our understanding of a normal serving of food has been grossly distorted. Today, what we consider a normal serving of food is actually one to two times more food than what a normal serving was in the past.

There is a reason why getting more food per serving is a problem. We all remember being told by our parents to "clean your plate" or that "children are starving in other places, so don't waste food" and "waste not want not." These petitions to not waste food are good advice, but as you'll see, not always necessary. Some of the more clever researchers in the world have been evaluating what happens when people are served larger serving sizes.[19] In one study, subjects were fed meals over a several week period. Unbeknownst to the subjects, the researchers served meals of different serving sizes. One serving size was one and a half times normal size and another two times the normal size. At the end of the study they measured how much food was consumed with each serving size. When the researchers served meals that were one and a half times the normal size, the subjects ate almost 500 calories more. When they served meals that were twice as large as normal, they ate 700 more calories. The larger the serving size they were served, the more they ate. On average, researchers have shown that when we are served large serving sizes compared to normal serving sizes we eat 30 to 50% more calories.[20] When we are served larger portions sizes we eat way more food and we feel like we've really gotten our money's worth.

Large serving sizes are the new food norm. We've come to expect large serving sizes when we dine out and even when we eat at home. Food trends show that restaurants all over the world are now serving large serving sizes.[21] Today, it's normal to be a little taken back if the meal we are served is not piled high on the plate. It's also normal for many people to dine out and split a meal or order a kid's meal. Today's kid's meals have enough food for adults. Not long ago on a speaking trip to Chicago I ordered an appetizer of lettuce wraps and a kid's meal pineapple pizza from a restaurant called California Pizza Kitchen. Either item by itself would have been plenty for my evening meal, and together they were enough for at least two people. These were the smallest servings I could see on their menu.

Bringing It All Together

If what I've been saying so far is true—if our unhealthy culture is to blame for our increasingly poor health, then there must be some direct evidence of how that culture has changed our choices and behaviors. We'll, we've just reviewed the evidence. The food industry serves us what we ask for, they want our money, and we want their food. By giving us what we want, our nutrition culture has changed dramatically. In the past 30 years we've added an additional 570 calories to our daily food intake. These extra calories have come from one of three places: 1) 1.1 extra eating occasions per day, mostly from snacking, 2) more food away from home, which has higher energy density in food and beverages, and/or 3) larger serving sizes. Of these three changes in our culture, which one explains the extra calories that we're eating? One researcher has indicated that 400 of these 570 calories we eat each day come from the extra snacking and the higher energy density foods.[6] We don't know the exact answer to this question, but we're learning more every day. What we do know is that our nutrition culture has changed in these three areas. This has resulted in poor health and excess weight among most Americans. Not only do we have a new food culture, we also have a new culture that discourages physical activity.

But don't get too discouraged with how much our culture has changed. With the right strategies, you'll soon be joining people like Amanda Wallace who have figured out how to create a healthy culture.

Island Native

My name is Amanda Wallace. I work as a sixth grade teacher in Boise, Idaho. Battling with my weight has always been a reality that I have had to deal with. What I didn't realize was that my weight could affect my ability to become pregnant. My husband and I were trying to have a child and it turned out that I was going to need to take some fertility medicine in order to get pregnant. I decided that I wanted to at least try to lose some weight and get healthy naturally. I thought, "If I can't be healthy before my kids are born, when will I learn a good lifestyle that I can teach them?"

Finding the right plan for eating healthy was really important to me. I decided to participate in my employer's wellness program. It really helped me get started by teaching me how to choose healthy alternatives, how to not eat too much and how to avoid high-calorie foods. After some initial success, I thought it would be a good idea to join an exercise group. A gym in my town was offering a boot camp. At first I felt really intimidated by gyms and thought that everyone would be staring at me. I definitely thought that during the first few classes, but after going regularly I started to feel comfortable with everyone in my group. Having a group to work out with helped keep me accountable and it helped me get acquainted with the gym and the equipment. As a person who has always had a hard time working out, I would recommend group exercise to everyone.

Lastly, without my husband, these changes wouldn't have been possible. He really supported me by cooking healthier foods at home. We stopped eating high-fat, high-sugar fast foods. If there was something I am most happy about with my changes it's that I can now buy "skinny jeans." It feels so good to look good and I don't want to go back to wearing my old clothes. For me, the hardest part of getting healthy was eating healthy. All I can say is, "Plan what you will eat the day before so that you won't choose the unhealthy convenient option." Now I feel like I can be a better mother because I know what it takes to be healthy.

When you think about it, these advancements are nothing short of miraculous. Each time I board an airplane, I think of my ancestors who pulled carts on foot or rode in wagons to cross the Great Plains. What took them months takes me hours and instead of walking, I sit. Any complaining about a delayed flight or travel inconvenience quickly goes away when I think about how good I have it. On one recent flight I watched the guy next to me get increasingly frustrated because his personal on-board television system only had 18 channels.

The benefits from these advancements are numerous, but they bring some challenges as well. Our society and culture have changed so quickly and the changes have been so drastic that we have not yet learned how to adapt. Like I said, 99.9% of all humans never had this lifestyle, so genetically, behaviorally and physically we are in new territory full of great benefits and dramatic detriments. This new territory involves an ever-evolving culture that we are pretty much making up as we go. Think, for example, of the changes to our language and vocabulary. Consider the origins of these words: couch potato, sedentary, fitness, obese, morbidly obese, type II diabetes, liposuction, aerobics, strength training, gym membership, treadmill…you get the idea. Do you think our ancestors would have a clue what any of these words mean? Pretend your great, great, grandmother (God rest her soul) stopped in for a visit and noticed your treadmill in the corner. How could you explain to her, in a way she would understand, why you spend 30 minutes walking on a device that doesn't take you anywhere? Just imagine her reaction when you explain how people use stationary bikes to pedal away only to go nowhere.

Our Ancestors Were Right

While doing some consulting for a large employer, I met Beatriz Donayre, a middle-aged administrative assistant originally from Peru. After being in the U.S. for about 15 years, she took a vacation and returned to Peru to visit her aging father. When she arrived at her father's village they embraced each other, and her father's first words were, "You are fat." And compared to everyone else in her family in Peru she was fat. Life in America had changed her, and not all the changes were good. Because she had grown accustomed to American food and became sedentary, she had gained around 45 pounds and developed type II diabetes. Her father, concerned about her health, took this moment to share some of his ageless wisdom with her, "Don't eat anything unless it comes from a tree or grows from the ground. And get rid of your car!"

These simple life lessons from a 102-year-old Peruvian villager are actually quite profound. In his simplicity, he was able to determine that a lifestyle based mostly on whole foods combined with regular physical activity results in a long, high quality life. Now, I'm not suggesting that you should get rid of your car, but his comments reveal a simple truth we can all learn from: the American lifestyle can hurt your health. Excess body fat and type II diabetes are indeed two of the possible negative side effects of our American way of life. Beatriz explained that her trip to Peru was a transforming experience. Fortunately, upon returning to the U.S. she succeeded in changing her lifestyle to better reflect her father's advice. She did not sell her car, but she did make time for regular, vigorous physical activity. Today she's no longer diabetic.

To further illustrate the problems associated with a sedentary lifestyle, let me tell you about the Pima Indians. Their native land is Arizona, but some have since crossed over into Mexico. These now separate groups are from the same original tribe and are genetically similar. They have both lived a traditional hunter-gatherer lifestyle for thousands of years, and the Pima Indians in Mexico continue to do so to this day. They are still physically active and they still eat the foods they've always eaten. The Pima Indians in Arizona on the other hand are far less physically active and have adopted a completely western diet. Shockingly, 38% of the Pima Indians in Arizona are type II diabetic. When you cross the border to Mexico, that number drops to just seven percent.[1] After thousands of years of living off the land and being physically active, the Pima Indians in Arizona have adopted a western lifestyle and now they are suffering the consequences. Their epidemic of diabetes is a result of their westernized lives and they personify the problem we are talking about in this chapter: Our culture has changed, we get less physical activity and now we suffer more chronic diseases.[2]

I'm the first to admit that the Pima Indians are an extreme example of how our western culture causes chronic diseases. For most of us, the impact of a sedentary lifestyle is much more subtle, but still just as deadly. Almost seven out of every 10 Americans will suffer and die from preventable chronic diseases such as diabetes, cancer and cardiovascular disease.[3] Even though these diseases take a long time to develop they begin when we start to live like Beatriz or the Arizona Pima Indians. We get jobs, we start families and we seem to get too busy to focus on our health. We spend more and more time sitting in the car, at a desk, and on the couch, and we have less and less free time for physical activity. For many, this results in weight gain, and for almost all, it results in worse health.

If you stop eating, you will quickly die. If you stop exercising completely, you could probably still live for years, maybe even decades before you die. Lack of exercise does not suddenly cause chronic disease—it takes years before the damage is done. This delay between the act—sedentary living—and the consequences—premature death and disease—only makes it harder for many people to be active. The delay can be decades, but it is only a delay, eventually the consequences are realized. With the passage of time our bodies slowly change, and we develop high blood pressure or high blood cholesterol. To make these problems go away, most Americans start taking pills, which only treats the symptoms, not the underlying problem. The real issue is not the high blood pressure or the high blood cholesterol; it's our unhealthy culture and specifically our lack of regular physical activity.

What We Have Become

I don't think any corporation that sells labor-saving devices ever thought that their products would cause harm. For example, the automobile industry has probably never wondered, "Hmm, if we create machines that will help people get from point A to point B do you think they will develop chronic diseases and die early?" The unhealthy culture we now live in is nothing more than an unfortunate side effect of our well-intended desires to reduce physical labor. In an effort to make money, businesses are more than happy to give customers what they want: "Buy Now, Pay Later" "What happens in Vegas, stays in Vegas" "Have it Your Way" "No Money Down" and so on. You don't even have to get out of your car because you can use the drive through to buy fast food, refill medications, deposit cash or even pick up your dry cleaning. You would think we would be ready to stand up and move around by the time we arrive home, but instead we open the garage door with the push of a button and we plop down in our favorite chair.

Honestly, labor-saving devices such as the garage door opener are only one of the many reasons why most Americans don't get very much physical activity. The nature of our work has also changed. Many people have very sedentary jobs. They spend the entire day driving a truck, sitting at a desk or working on the computer. In the past, many jobs involved physical activity and some still do, but today most jobs in America involve sitting. Even the farmers who grow our food will spend much of their days sitting on equipment as they work the earth. Pressure to keep up with the Jones' causes many of us to work more and more hours, which means more time sitting down. Americans work more hours per week than any other country in the world, and most of these hours are spent sitting.

In addition to demanding work schedules and pressure to earn more money, there are other factors in society that keep us from being physically active. Some people live in neighborhoods or communities with high rates of crime, which make it dangerous to walk around. Others live in neighborhoods where there are no sidewalks or safe places to walk or jog. Naturally, most of our communities are designed to accommodate automobile traffic, not pedestrians. Most suburbs are designed for people who commute every day. A car or public transportation is a must if you want any basics like groceries or medical attention. We drive—not walk—to work, school and the grocery store. The No Child Left Behind law has forced many schools to reduce physical education classes so they can devote more time to studying.[4] Some schools have even stopped having recess because it cuts into valuable learning time. Many buildings have stairwells that are poorly lit, inconvenient and sometimes just plain scary. Elevators are built in the center of buildings and are designed to be convenient. After all, it's easier to take the elevator than the stairs. The design of our buildings, communities, schools and neighborhoods have been altered in a way that supports minimal physical activity.

Inside The Aldana Home

When I was a boy, computer games were just beginning to appear. There used to be an electronic tennis game called Pong. It had two dials used to bounce a ball of light between two sides of the screen. It was awesome. Recently, I showed this game to my 15-year-old son. He was polite enough to acknowledge my sincere nostalgia for the game, but quick to point out the obvious fact that compared to the games he plays today, Pong is one of the most boring games ever invented.

Today, my children play computer games that defy imagination. The boys in the neighborhood will get together and play, but instead of running around in the front yard, they will sit on two or three different computers and play games. Most often, they don't even come over, they simply sit at home and use headphones and microphones to interactively play and communicate with one another. One day I was watching my son play one of these games and asked who he was playing with. He was one of three people on his team. The other two were a new friend in Portugal and a friend from Malaysia. Three 15-year-old boys from three different countries playing an electronic game that put Pong to shame.

These games are so fun they can become addictive. It didn't take long for my wife and I to see that playing these games could quickly become an unhealthy pastime. We had to institute the two-hour screen time rule. This is how it works: each child gets to spend two hours in front of a screen each day (screen time includes television, movies, electronic games and anything on the computer). After two hours their time is up. When they're done for the day they must find something else to do. In the beginning, they acted as if we had chopped off an arm or a leg, but soon they discovered that there were other things to do and even (gasp!) great books to read and delicious meals to prepare. One study showed that parents who implement rules limiting screen time reduce children's screen time by 70%.[5]

For many years, public health officials were worried about the amount of time people were spending sitting in front of a television. Today, time spent in front of the television is only one way we spend our free time being sedentary. Children between the ages of one and six spend an average of two hours a day watching television.[6] It's worse among teenagers. They just don't watch television, but they also play video games and watch movies. A national survey of teenagers recently found that the average teenager spends almost eight hours in front of electronic screens per day.[5] This is in addition to spending approximately eight hours every day in school. Unless children and teenagers are getting regular physical activity at school, it is very unlikely that they are being even remotely active sitting in front of electronic screens. In fact, one of the best predictors of fitness is the amount of time spent in front of an electronic screen. As the amount of time goes up, the level of fitness goes down.[7]

Even the ability to participate in organized sports has changed. Unless you live in an area with relatively small schools the only real chance a child has to participate in school sports is if they spend many years playing in expensive sports clubs. There was a time when children could participate in many different sports in school. Today, however, only the best and most competitive youth will make sports teams. In many ways, high school sports have become like college sports. Only the affluent have the resources that allow their children to participate in organized sports. Today children are attracted to a variety of electronic games and activities that require no physical activity and often fill free time with sedentary activities that would have otherwise been filled with sports.

It's no surprise that our children are unfit and rapidly becoming obese. Not long ago, it was common for moms and dads to go to the front door and yell, "Kids, it's time to come in for dinner." Today parents often have to plead with their children, "Kids, you need to go outside and play." My, how things have changed.

The tobacco industry makes money selling a product that kills people. Of course, sedentary living is not like the tobacco industry because there is no actual product being manufactured. But like the tobacco industry, there are many industries that benefit financially from our sedentary ways. Health care providers, pharmaceutical companies, dialysis centers, insurance companies and many others make substantial amounts of money treating the diseases that are caused by our sedentary ways. In essence, many in our society today make a very good living on the new culture we have created. Sitting in front of computer screens and in our cars all day dramatically reduces our physical activity and eventually causes the need to treat chronic diseases that support so many companies.

In 2001, the Segway company introduced the new Segway, a self-balancing electric vehicle. A technological marvel, the Segway integrated a variety of sensors and electronics to make guiding and operating the vehicle as natural as walking. It is truly an amazing device, one that reduces the need for walking. Just like the automobile, the Segway does an outstanding job of completely eliminating the need to do any physical work. That's good for saving time and avoiding the need to sweat, but ultimately it reduces our level of fitness, prevents our cardiovascular system from growing stronger and eventually leads to the development chronic diseases. The Segway removes our biological need to be active and is just one more example of how technology is working against our biological need to move around.

We no longer grow our own food. This is not a bad thing but it is a change. Few of us use our physical strength to plant, grow and harvest the food we eat. We let others do this work. Digging in the dirt to grow fruits and vegetables for consumption is almost a dying art and further evidence that our culture has undergone some dramatic changes.

To make up for our lack of physical activity we have created a multi-billion-dollar fitness industry with fitness classes, exercise machinery and personalized training. We have spinning, cycling, aerobics, interval training, weight training and Zumba (for those who don't know about Zumba, it's a Latin dance/martial arts inspired fitness program). Zumba classes are exciting and just saying the word Zumba is fun. None of this existed a century ago because most people got enough physical activity in their everyday lives.

Percentage Of Adults Who Get Enough Exercise To Reap The Benefits[8]

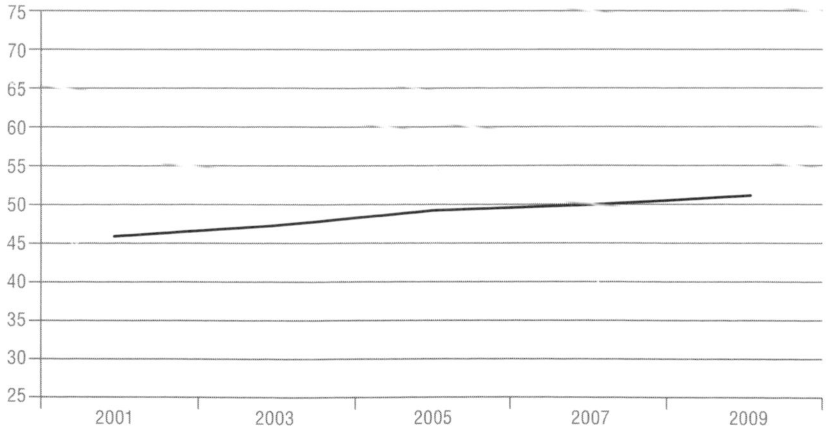

Little of this information is news to most of us. We've all known that our world has changed. Despite the changes in our culture and the known benefits associated with being physically active the number of adults getting regular physical activity has remained remarkably flat.

Over the last decade, the number of adults who get enough physical activity to reap the benefits has only increased slightly. Since the 1940s, the amount of physical activity Americans get is relatively unchanged. This graph shows the biggest increases in almost 100 years have just recently occurred and even these increases are very small.

Does It Really Matter If I Exercise?

Our unhealthy American culture forces many of us to be inactive. Not moving is a very real and normal part of life. After all, most people spend one-third of their entire lives asleep, tucked between the bed sheets. There's not a lot of exercise occurring when we're sleeping, and that is perfectly okay. The problems arise when we spend almost all of our waking hours not moving around.

Remember, for the past 100,000 years humans have been doing a lot of physical activity, so our bodies have adapted to those demands. The very act of moving involves the heart, lungs, brain, and numerous vessels, muscles, bones, joints and nerves, just to mention a few. Each of these body parts has become highly efficient and skilled in its role because its had a lot of practice. The bodies we have today are actually the result of 100,000 years of modifications, improvements and enhancements needed to function in a world that required lots of physical activity. Our bodies have been built to move and suddenly we're telling them to sit. The world our bodies have been designed for no longer exists for many of us and therein lies the problem. We've created a different society where we no longer need to be as active and so our bodies suffer.

When you exercise, your muscles exert forces on your bones as you strain under the added pressure. The bones sense this strain and slowly deposit more bone in order to prepare for the next time. Exercise makes your bones stronger. So, what if you don't exercise? No exercise means no muscle strain which means no bone strain which means no added deposits. The result is osteoporosis. In a very real way, no physical activity can cause osteoporosis.[9]

Of course, there are even more exercise benefits you should be aware of. When you exercise, your body does a good job of controlling your blood pressure. Blood pressure stays normal because your blood vessels have become accustomed to dilating and contracting as your heart beats harder during exercise. Exercise causes your blood vessels to remain flexible which helps keep your blood pressure normal. So, what if you don't exercise? Your heart doesn't work hard and the vessels rarely have to respond to big changes in pressure. They actually get accustomed to not flexing and they become stiff. The result is arteriosclerosis which leads to high blood pressure. Since the vessels are no longer flexible, your blood pressure increases. Therefore, lack of regular physical activity usually results in hypertension. And as you probably know, high blood pressure is a cause of heart disease, stroke and kidney failure.

Let's talk about your heart. Just like other muscles in your body, your heart has to work harder during exercise. To keep beating hard, your heart needs a really good supply of oxygen and nutrients. No one knows exactly how, but when you exercise your heart actually develops additional capillaries to make sure the blood has easy access to the heart muscle. This increased blood supply has two effects.[10] First, it dramatically lowers your chances of having a heart attack. Second, if you are unfortunate enough to have one, the amount of damage that occurs to your heart is greatly reduced. This is because all the exercise you did actually created additional blood vessels, which help keep some blood flowing, even after an artery gets blocked. So, what if you don't exercise? Your risk of having a heart attack goes way up, and if you do happen to have one the damage is significantly worse, often resulting in cardiac failure and death.[11]

Exercise is particularly beneficial for women because it can help prevent breast cancer. Women who exercise have less body fat, they produce less female hormones like estrogen and they have a slightly improved immune system. Each of these benefits has the potential to affect how the body controls or stops the growth of abnormal cells. If you don't exercise, you don't get these benefits and you have a much higher risk of getting breast cancer.[12]

Every time you eat, you consume energy. All that energy has to go somewhere. For most Americans, the energy we've eaten that exceeds what we need each day gets stored as fat. Most Americans are storing a lot of excess energy because we eat way more calories than we burn. Physical activity is the single biggest resource we have to burn off the excess energy we consume. No exercise, no calorie burn. It's no coincidence that the obesity epidemic in the U.S. is directly linked to our lack of physical activity and poor diet. We consume more calories than ever and we exercise less. No wonder we gain weight.

This excess energy collection has a darker, more serious consequence to it as well. All of your muscles and organs need energy to function. And in order for energy to get from the blood into the cells of your body, the energy has to have a special escort. This escort is called insulin. When we eat too much of the wrong kinds of food a large amount of digested calories—now in the form of sugar—gets released into our blood stream. There is so much blood sugar that the insulin can't keep up with demand so the excess sugar backs up in the blood stream.

Physical activity plays a critical role in this story.[13] When we don't get much physical activity, we don't use our muscles much. In essence, this is what sedentary muscles are saying: "Hey you escort dudes, go ahead and take the day off. We won't be needing your services because we're not doing anything today." After hearing this day after day, the escorts change a bit and some forget how to do their job. In reality, your body will either stop producing enough insulin or your cells will stop recognizing it. Either way, the energy can't get into the cells which means it gets backed up into the bloodstream. Having high blood sugar is a sure sign that either your diet is dumping too much sugar into your body too quickly or your muscles are inactive and no longer have the need for much insulin, or both. The risk of type II diabetes goes way up for those who are sedentary, and if you are type II diabetic, it's very difficult to live a long, healthy life. But if this is you, don't lose hope because as you'll read later, it's not too late to change.

In addition to the physical benefits, regular exercise also offers benefits to your emotional well-being. There is scientific evidence that exercise can increase the levels of several mood-enhancing chemicals that get released in your brain. Regular exercise increases the release of endorphins, which are the hormones that make you feel good. We all need a little more of that in our lives, don't we? On top of boosting your mood, exercise also reduces your stress hormones and helps relieve the stress you are already feeling. As the stress hormones in your blood decrease, your muscles actually relax more completely. Exercise also increases body temperature, which has a calming effect. As a result, people who exercise are usually able to sleep better. Without these chemical, muscle and temperature changes, you may not be getting quality sleep.[14]

Besides better sleep, using exercise to reduce your stress can also help you overcome sadness, anxiety, anger, depression and feelings of hopelessness. So let's ask the question again: what if you don't exercise? Well, you could end up being a stressed out, exhausted, miserable, angry, depressed person who really needs a big hug.

How about clearing your mind? During exercise, a different portion of your brain becomes more active which means the other parts get a rest. Exercise can actually shift the focus away from the problems, worries or tasks you have been thinking about, and put the focus on the part of the brain that's needed for exercise. Some research has shown that fresh ideas, answers to problems or new ways of thinking are more likely to come to us when we take a break from our daily routine and engage in some form of physical activity. Think of what we miss when we're sedentary. We may be preventing ourselves from tapping into our brain's full potential to help us be more creative and productive.

The List Of Benefits Grows

During the summer of 2005 I wrote *The Culprit & The Cure*. For this book, I reviewed all the current science that looked at the benefits of getting regular exercise. There was a lot of research to look at and I discussed every benefit that was backed by strong evidence. Some would like to claim that exercise can heal or prevent everything, but that's simply not the case. Exercise has a dramatic impact on our health and quality of life, but I prefer to share the benefits for which there is solid scientific research. Since my last review in 2005, the science has been able to show additional benefits for both men and women.

It's hard to watch television these days and not see commercials promoting drugs for the treatment of erectile dysfunction in men. One of the more popular drugs for treating erectile dysfunction is called Viagra. Originally it was developed to treat hypertension and angina (heart pain). Early trials with the drug showed that it had very little effect on hypertension, however, patients reported that the drug had an interesting side effect. Their problems with erectile dysfunction disappeared when they took Viagra. It is ironic that one of the most profitable drugs ever taken to market was discovered by complete accident when it failed to treat hypertension, but was accidentally discovered to be a treatment for erectile dysfunction. Erectile dysfunction is a disease of the blood vessels. Heart disease is also a disease of the blood vessels. If exercise is such a good treatment for heart disease because it helps improve blood flow and strengthen the heart, why wouldn't exercise also be a good treatment for erectile dysfunction? That is exactly the same question that researchers have been investigating. One of the additional benefits of regular exercise is that your blood vessels become more fit. Blood vessels contract and expand better and help blood flow in both arteries and veins, helping to supply important nutrients to your cells. When patients with erectile dysfunction start exercising regularly their condition disappears. There are now a variety of good studies showing that one of the most effective treatments for erectile dysfunction is regular physical activity—no pills required.[15]

If you are a male and you have cardiovascular disease chances are very good that you may also have erectile dysfunction. The opposite is also true, if you are a male with erectile dysfunction chances are you also have cardiovascular disease.[16] Erectile dysfunction and cardiovascular disease appeared together in many cases because they are simply symptoms of the same problem: an unhealthy lifestyle that includes very little physical activity. Some have even suggested that the presence of erectile dysfunction is a very good predictor or risk factor for cardiovascular disease.[17]

Exercise has now also been shown to decrease the risk of developing chronic mental conditions such as Parkinson's disease and Alzheimer's. If you look at an individual's lifestyle including good nutrition, regular physical activity, social support and other factors, there is more and more outstanding research showing that the onset of dementia is strongly correlated with these lifestyle choices.[18] Just like cardiovascular disease and erectile dysfunction, blood vessels are also involved in dementia. The build-up of proteins and plaques in the vessels of the brain cause these forms of dementia. Once again, there is a growing body of scientific research that has connected our unhealthy culture and lifestyle with the onset of chronic diseases, including dementia.

Prevention, Arrest and Reversal

One of the most exciting discoveries over the last few years is that some of the chronic diseases that inflict humans can be prevented, arrested (that is, they don't get any worse) or even reversed. These discoveries are critically important because they tell us that it's never too late to change. It would appear from the studies of type II diabetes and cardiovascular disease that those with these diseases can actually reverse the damage that has been done by an unhealthy lifestyle. Often, people feel that they are too old or that it's too hard for them to change and that change for them is not possible. There is now very good evidence that for those who are willing to adopt and maintain a healthy lifestyle these conditions can be reversed. The studies tell us that despite what people think, it is possible to teach old dogs new tricks. For those with cardiovascular disease, the best evidence and program for reversal has been written by Dr. Caldwell Esselstyn and explained in his book *Prevent and Reverse Heart Disease: The Revolutionary, Scientifically Proven, Nutrition-Based Cure.* I highly recommend this book for those who are struggling with this disease.

Those who are struggling with type II diabetes have even better news. Reversal of the disease is possible, as long as the disease is still relatively new. I conducted two studies evaluating the impact of a healthy lifestyle change program on working adults. Those employees who were diabetic or pre-diabetic were invited to participate in an employee wellness program targeting diabetes.[19–20] We discovered that there were 35 employees at this worksite who were pre-diabetic or diabetic but did not know it. We invited all 35 and their spouses or significant others to participate in a worksite diabetes program conducted by a nurse and a local health intern. They learned about good nutrition and regular exercise and even had opportunities to get exercise while at work. After six months, 22 of the 35 diabetic employees were no longer diabetic. Six months is good, but I'm more impressed with data that is longer than six months. Sometimes people make healthy lifestyle choices in the short term, but after a while they succumb to the pressures of an unhealthy culture and revert back to their old, unhealthy ways. We evaluated the same 35 employees after one and a half years and were delighted to see that 22 of the 35 were still diabetes free. When we measured their blood glucose and other diabetes markers, it was clear they had experienced reversal of a chronic disease that if left unchecked would shorten their lives between seven and 14 years. Of course, if there were 22 employees who changed that means there were 13 who did not. These 13 were unable to change their behaviors, they were unable to make regular physical activity a part of their daily lives and they are likely still suffering from this debilitating disease today.

Not all cases of type II diabetes can be reversed. With type II diabetes the pancreas, which produces insulin, actually gets destroyed over time. The longer you live with type II diabetes the more permanent damage is done to the pancreas. The ability to reverse this disease is very much dependent upon how long you've had the disease. After decades of suffering from diabetes and using multiple medications for many years, it becomes much more difficult to reverse the condition. Like most things, the earlier you begin the better.

With diabetes, once the pancreas has been destroyed it is impossible to get it to grow back. But with cardiovascular disease, tissue is not destroyed. With this disease, our arteries get blocked by fats, cholesterol and plaque that actually form alongside and within the artery wall. Reversal of this condition can happen regardless of how long you've had it. When you adopt a lifestyle that includes regular physical activity and a healthy diet, you actually stop the process that is causing the arteries to be blocked in the first place. Unless the heart itself has been damaged, changing to a healthy lifestyle can reverse the cardiovascular disease process. The best evidence that a chronic disease can be reversed comes from the studies on cardiovascular disease. Reversal of cancer is an entirely different story.

Regular physical activity has a powerful impact on the prevention of both breast cancer and colon cancer. With a healthy lifestyle, the odds of getting these two types of cancer are greatly reduced. Regular physical activity is very effective at preventing these cancers from ever occurring, however, once these cancers or any other cancer for that matter start, the ability of regular exercise and a healthy diet to arrest the cancer (stop it from getting worse) or reversing it is unlikely. When you actually develop cancer, all the healthy living in the world is unlikely to have much effect on the growth of abnormal cancer cells. But, despite the expense, our current health care system is extremely good at treating cancers once they're in place. And just like cancer, once dementia sets in we're past the window of opportunity where prevention will have much effect. There is no evidence that regular physical activity can reverse dementia.

Finally, when we talk about prevention, arrest and reversal of chronic diseases we need to add death to this discussion. The death rate in the U.S. hasn't changed for a very long time. It's still one per person! Everyone who has ever walked on the earth has a date with the Grim Reaper. Death is inevitable. The only part of this story we don't know is when and how we will pass away. Several very large studies have looked at the impact of sedentary living on premature death and the results are pretty conclusive. If you don't move around much, you are almost twice as likely to die early. When combined with a poor diet, those who are sedentary will die about 10 to 20 years earlier than they would have if they had made better lifestyle choices.[21]

Since most people have unhealthy diets and are sedentary, it's not unreasonable to suggest that most Americans are dying 10 to 20 years earlier than they should. For those who are physically active, don't smoke and have a healthy diet it's also reasonable to suggest that they are enjoying 10 to 20 years of extra life and that these extra years of life are high quality. No one wants to spend 10 to 20 extra years suffering from chronic diseases. In fact, one of the main reasons this book is so important is because it provides the pathway to help people enjoy 10 to 20 years of extra, high-quality life. Death is inevitable for everyone but why not put it off as long as possible?

There is so much about the benefits of regular exercise that we do not understand. Scientists all over the world are carefully studying how regular physical activity impacts our lives. I have a feeling that as the research on physical activity continues we will discover even more benefits associated with having an active lifestyle.

Be More Active Today

To prevent chronic diseases, the current exercise guidelines recommend that all adults do 30 to 60 minutes of moderate-intensity exercise (five days per week) or 20 to 60 minutes of vigorous-intensity exercise (three days per week).[22] Moderate-intensity physical activity means working hard enough to raise your heart rate and break a sweat, yet still being able to carry on a conversation. To lose weight or maintain weight loss, 60 to 90 minutes of daily physical activity may be necessary.

We've had these recommendations for a long time, yet over half of all the adults in the United States don't get the minimal amount of exercise to reap the benefits. How much more exercise does the typical person have to get in order to start getting the benefits? Can people really change their lifestyles and become more active? How long does it take for them to start realizing the benefits?

I spent almost 20 years as a professor doing research on the benefits of a healthy lifestyle. With all that I had learned and discovered I left academia a few years ago to start the behavior change company called WellSteps. WellSteps provides wellness programs for employers who are trying to improve the health of their employees. I used all of the information, tools and best research to create programs that help people adopt and maintain healthy behaviors—like regular physical activity. To show you how it's possible to become more physically active and enjoy all the benefits of being active, I want to share some of the results we published not long ago. One particular wellness client of mine includes employees who are engineers, staff workers and sewage treatment specialists. After two years of participating in our wellness programs we reported the results.[23]

Of the 472 employees at this company, the average employee was getting 120 minutes of exercise a week at the beginning of the program; that's less than the recommended amount of 150 to 300 minutes per week. After one year, they increased their exercise minutes per week to 198 minutes. This was a dramatic improvement from where they started and represents a huge improvement in fitness for this company. However, 12 months is a short amount of time, so we did another evaluation after two years. After 24 months, the average employee was exercising 193 minutes per week. They had also increased the number of days they were exercising per week from 2 to 3.2 days per week. With the right tools and right strategies and with peer support, we have demonstrated that it is possible for large numbers of sedentary individuals to make exercise a regular part of their lives. When this is combined with the employees' improvements in nutrition, we can easily determine that they are all well on their way to preventing chronic diseases and living long, high quality lives. The average age of these individuals was 46, so it appears once again that you can teach old dogs new tricks.

To prevent chronic diseases, the current exercise guidelines recommend that all adults do 30 to 60 minutes of moderate-intensity exercise (five days per week) or 20 to 60 minutes of vigorous-intensity exercise (three days per week).

This is one of many examples of how people who live in a culture that does not encourage regular physical activity can create an alternate culture that supports an active lifestyle. These employees have been able to maintain their physical activity patterns for at least two years and I'm confident that they are now experiencing the benefits and will continue to be active for the rest of their lives.

Changing Our Couch Potato Culture

For 100,000 years, we labored and toiled to provide food, shelter and clothing for ourselves and our families. Today, we provide the same needs for ourselves and families by sitting in our cars, sitting at our desks or working with the assistance of labor-saving devices. In the same way that our diets have changed, we have abandoned much of our ancient ways of being active. This cultural shift away from a life of physical activity is most obvious among our native populations who now live sedentary lives and eat westernized foods. All of our technological advances, labor-saving devices and modern modes of transportation have turned us into a sedentary population. All of these changes could be considered an unfortunate side effect of our modern society. Unfortunately, our ancient bodies are unable to adapt to life without regular physical activity. Not enough time has passed for us to adapt to this new way of living. Adaptations can occur, but it takes tens of thousands of years. Maybe 10,000 years from now the human body will be able to be mostly sedentary and not develop chronic diseases, but for now you and I are stuck. We're stuck with ancient bodies in a modern world. No pills, potions or spas will be able to protect us from the health consequences caused by a lack of regular physical activity. What will protect us is a new culture within a culture where we enjoy all the benefits of our modern civilization while at the same time providing our bodies with the physical activity they need to function properly. But, as you are about to learn, the forces working against your desires to have a healthy lifestyle aren't going away any time soon.

Island Native

My name is Ted Overcash and I work as an equipment operator in Harrisburg, Pennsylvania. What really shocked me about my health was that I did not feel sick or bad at all. I guess I wasn't really sick, but I could have gotten really sick. I found out I was pre-diabetic through a health screening at work. I was terrified, I had no idea. I had a brother who lost a leg to diabetes, but I thought I had been "spared" because I didn't have any symptoms. Along with having pre-diabetes, I had high blood pressure and high cholesterol. I learned that I needed to change. Thankfully, my doctor didn't just prescribe me some medicine, but he helped teach me how to live a better life.

The first thing to go from my diet was fast food. The second, and probably the hardest, was my Dr. Pepper. After I gave that up, it was easy to stop adding sugar to my coffee and eating fried chicken (one of my favorite foods). I started eating more healthy foods like salad.

At work I say to myself, "An object in motion stays in motion." For me, this means if I take time to sit down and lollygag, then I will have a hard time getting back up and working. It is my way of staying active at work and it helps me get motivated to walk up a few extra flights of stairs after work. Another habit of mine that I am working hard to quit is smoking. I used to smoke two packs a day and now I smoke half a pack a day. I have been using my motivation to stay active and eat healthy to help me quit smoking.

One of the things I care about most in my life is my family. These changes have primarily been because I want to live for them. I have a new grandson and I want nothing more than to take him hunting. I don't want to take him with a missing leg or huffing and puffing. I want to take him and enjoy it myself. Without these changes I know I wouldn't be able to do it. Aside from wanting to be there for my family, these changes have helped me feel great and look great. You can't beat fitting back into your clothes from high school. If there is one thing you can learn from me I would say it would be, "Don't give up. It is worth it in the long run, and if you don't have good health, you have nothing."

CHAPTER 7

Win, Win, Lose

AS YOU AND I STRUGGLE TO HAVE OPTIMAL HEALTH WE WILL HAVE TO OVERCOME THE POWERFUL CULTURAL FACTORS THAT INFLUENCE OUR EATING AND EXERCISE BEHAVIORS. Our toxic food and exercise culture is so engrained into our everyday life that only the most dedicated are able to escape its influences. These influences are not going away anytime soon and researchers estimate that by the year 2030, 51% of all adults in the U.S. will be obese.[1] Before we talk specifically about how people actually win this battle for better health it is important that you understand precisely what you are up against. Be warned, some of you are not going to like what I'm about to talk about in this chapter. It is not my intention to offend, but merely to paint a picture about how we have arrived at this precarious place. Anytime you talk about someone's profession or about politics people are bound to get emotional. I have spent my entire adult life trying to figure out how to help people achieve good health. I, along with others, have come to a clear conclusion that our unhealthy culture is the outcome of self-serving interests that have taken precedence over public health. I'm not talking about the overt nastiness that pervades the tobacco industry; I'm talking about individuals and politicians who, in the course of trying to do the right thing, have created unintended consequences in the form of chronic disease, early death and the obesity epidemic. Once you have a clear understanding of how we have arrived in this situation the clouds will lift and the pathway to better health will become obvious. You will ultimately be able to see why the only long-term solution will require you to create and live in a new culture of health.

Although there are professional and governmental agencies created with the intent to help you and I have healthy, long lives, these groups are not coming to the rescue. They fully understand how severe this problem has become and many of them really do care, but their help is severely limited because they are conflicted. They are not entirely committed to your health because their allegiance is shared with organizations and companies that are more interested in making money than helping you stay healthy. Because they are conflicted, they are by default ineffective and can even make it difficult for you and me to be healthy.

The Nutrition Priesthood

Can you think of any group of individuals or organization that has direct responsibility to ensure that Americans have a healthy diet? Is there a profession that has been charged with advancing public health and nutrition? Actually, there is. This group is the American Dietetics Association, now known as the Academy of Nutrition and Dietetics. This professional organization represents 70,000 registered dietitians devoted to applying the principles of food and nutrition to health. In a very real sense, they are the guardians of all things nutritional, standing watch over the nutrition industry, government policies and public health initiatives that impact our health. For years, registered dietitians have helped improve public health by educating people, working with patients who have nutritional needs, and assisting schools, worksites and communities to improve their nutrition. This group also includes food scientists who have developed methods to keep our food safe. All this work is commendable. However, there is a much darker side to what this organization has become and though you may have never heard of them, your nutrition and health is under their influence.

For almost 50 years, this group has been helping its members become the nation's food and nutrition leaders. They have positioned themselves as the ultimate source of nutrition information and science—the "high priests of human nutrition," with a level of authority that could be considered nutrition priesthood. Anyone outside of the priesthood is a heretic, an apostate or a false prophet who should be silenced. I don't blame them for protecting their turf; that's a pretty standard survival tactic. The problem arises when the priesthood itself has become corrupt. I know these are some pretty strong words and perhaps I'm being unfair, but consider the following.

As the members of the Academy of Nutrition and Dietetics have been controlling and influencing the nutrition of Americans, the typical American diet has changed in such a way that we now have the fattest population in world history. The prevalence of diabetes has never been higher and will continue to get worse. So, while the nation's leading nutrition professionals have been guarding and protecting our citizens, the health of those very citizens has gotten to a point where it has never been worse. In a very real way, this organization has at best been a silent participant and at worst a direct cause of our now toxic food culture.

The problem is quite simple. The nutrition professionals in the United States who are part of the Academy are conflicted. Their allegiance has been divided between protecting the health of Americans and serving the food industry, from which they gain jobs and financial support. This is just one example of the win, win, lose arrangements that have direct control over your health. The Academy wins because they get money from the food industry, the food industry wins because they get the endorsement and support of the Academy, and you the consumer loses. You lose because the nutrition experts in collaboration with the food industry have declared that there is "no such thing as a bad food: all foods are good. Moderation is the key." My personal favorite is "it's all about personal responsibility." To be sure, you lose time and time again because many foods are allowed to be promoted as something they are not—healthy. You lose because the food industry is allowed to use confusing labels and outright deception to get you to buy their products. You lose because salt, sugar and fat permeate most processed and fast foods and nutrition professionals simply look the other way because they do not want to bite the hand that feeds them.

The Academy gets direct financial contributions from the largest food corporations in the world, including General Mills, Kellogg's, Mars, Coca-Cola, Pepsico, the National Dairy Council and the Hershey Corporation. Go to any of the Academy's national conferences and you will be instantly smothered by advertisements and promotions from food manufacturers who not only pay money to be at the conference, but also seek the blessing of the Academy. The relationship between the nutrition professionals and the food industry is extremely close. In fact, this relationship can be compared to the one that exists between the bankers and government banking regulators. Banking professionals who understand the nuances of the banking world take jobs as regulators within government while government banking regulators often take jobs in the private banking sector. It doesn't take long for the bankers to have tremendous influence over the regulatory process and for you, the consumer, to be taken advantage of. As directed by congress, bankers are asked to serve as regulators of their own industry. It's like a fox being asked to guard the hen house—the opportunities for abuse are enormous.

The revolving door within the nutrition industry functions very much the same way. Nutrition experts who have been trained by the Academy often take jobs in the food industry. Likewise, food industry experts belong to the Academy and also take jobs in federal government. It doesn't take long for the food industry to have influence over national food policy. Nutrition professionals that should be protecting public health are "in bed" with the food industry and are hesitant to do anything that will harm that relationship. This cozy relationship has caused nutrition professionals to compromise their mission to improve public health. The fact that public obesity and diabetes have never been worse is proof that the guardians of our health are asleep at the job. Somebody needs to wake them up or fire them. How can any member of the Academy look at our current state of health and think that everything in the nutrition world is just fine?

Two Masters

As we go about our daily lives, it may be hard to see how all of this discussion about the food industry and the nutrition Academy impacts each of us, but it does. The relationship between the food industry and nutrition professionals gets even more complicated when the federal government is involved. Every time I get on an airplane and travel at 35,000 feet I'm thankful for government employees at the FAA who help keep me safe. In fact, I feel safer traveling high above the earth than I do traveling on the road. This is just one area in which the federal government does an outstanding job of keeping us safe and enhancing our lives. I have a long list of wonderful benefits our federal government provides, but of course I also have a long list of things the federal government does that drives me crazy.

Despite all the good intentions of those who create our laws and regulations, by the time the regulations get to us they have a very different result. Much of the blame for our poor health can be placed on the federal government, which just like the nutrition Academy, has become conflicted.

Just like the nutrition professionals, the federal government is also guilty of trying to serve two masters when it makes nutrition recommendations and regulations. The federal government serves the larger U.S. economy while also trying to serve the federal mandate to improve public health. Meat producers, farms and the food industry provide good paying jobs. Jobs provide money for individuals who help keep the economy running. The conflict arises when the federal government tries to serve two purposes that are in direct conflict with one another. You see the direct result of this conflict every single day; it determines what you eat, and ultimately it determines whether or not you experience chronic disease and premature death. It might be hard to imagine how this could be possible, but let me share the evidence with you.

Take a look at the ingredients of just about any food you have recently eaten. Chances are pretty good that it contains high-fructose corn syrup (HFCs). This is basically added sugar that comes from corn. This extra sugar is in your food because we like foods that are sweet and high-fructose corn syrup is way cheaper than real, plain sugar. It's cheaper because the federal government subsidizes farmers who grow corn. Because of the federal subsidies, farmers can grow a lot of corn and still make good profits. This keeps the cost of high-fructose corn syrup very low—so low that food producers can now add this sweetener to just about every food at almost no added cost. Foods that used to contain sugar now contain high-fructose corn syrup because it's much cheaper to produce. This is another win, win, lose scenario that has a direct impact on your health and quality of life. Farmers win because they get good prices for the crops they grow. The food industry wins because their products are less expensive to make and because of the added sugar they know that you will buy more. You, the consumer, lose because the top source of calories in the U.S. today is from high-fructose corn syrup. A well-intended federal policy that is loved by farmers and the food industry has had a disastrous impact on our health. New Testament wisdom suggests that whenever one attempts to serve two masters somebody loses.[2] Much of the excess body weight we are gaining can be linked to the misguided actions of our federal government.

The health of our children is also impacted by the conflicted food regulations that come from our federal government. It was a fantastic idea back in the 1930s to take surplus food commodities that would have otherwise gone to waste and make them available to school children. The surplus food commodities gradually turned into the national school lunch program, which provides meals for children across the United States. What started as a very good idea has gradually morphed into something very different. Food corporations aggressively lobbied congress to purchase processed foods instead of just raw food commodities. Rather than buying excess fresh produce, schools were able to buy frozen cheese pizza, tater tots and many other highly processed foods. Once this door was open, food manufacturers pounced on the opportunity that would allow the federal government to buy their foods for the youth of America. It didn't take long for the first vending machines to pop up in schools, but congress wanted to protect the school lunch program so they made a rule that vending machines could not be in the same cafeteria where USDA food is being served (as if a distance of 10 feet would be sufficient to keep kids from buying Dr. Pepper instead of government-purchased pork). Almost instantly, vending machines began appearing in schools across America because the vendors could make huge profits. The schools could also make extra money, and the students had access to candy and soda all day long—another win, win, lose arrangement. Today, vending machines in schools provide hundreds of millions of dollars in revenue for school districts and the availability of highly processed foods in school cafeterias has become the new norm. Our federal government, under the continual pressure from food industry lobbyists and with the blessing of our nation's nutrition professionals, has created a system that is helping to produce the fattest population in human history.

Did you know that pizza is a vegetable? It is according to the complex rules and regulations of the USDA who has been greatly influenced by those who stand to make money selling pizza. Because of the tomato paste that is on pizza, it can be classified as a vegetable and because it is considered to be a vegetable, it helps schools meet the daily fruit and vegetable requirements they must serve to students. Mega food corporations like ConAgra and Schwan spent millions lobbying congress to keep pizza designated as a vegetable. Their money was well spent; congress caved to their demands, jobs were maintained, re-elections secured and vegetable designations preserved. Once again, we see win, win, lose in action. Every time a threat to corporate profits appears, the food industry unleashes a wave of lobbying efforts to control congress, and because nutrition professionals are also beholden to the same financial pressures they fail to intervene to protect public health.

I have been before congress to talk about these very issues. I very quickly learned that what you and I view as a clear conflict of interest is just business as usual for members of congress. When I bring up the ability of the food industry to influence legislative and regulatory processes, the politicians I talk to quickly go on the defensive. A typical response goes something like this: "How dare you accuse us of accepting money for political influence. If you think for a moment that our decisions are influenced by donations you don't know us. The money does nothing to influence the laws we pass." Without exception, members of congress will deny that special interests or lobbyists or the money they provide for campaigning influence the process. And yet, if this is the case why do corporations spend billions of dollars to hire lobbyists and finance election campaigns? Either the members of congress have an alternate version of reality or the food corporations of America are run by idiots who waste valuable profits on a useless effort to influence the legislative process. I believe corporations are fully aware of how valuable their lobbying efforts are. The money they spend to influence the political process is one of the best business investments they can make. They are well-funded and you are not. They help keep people in office with their financial support, and you (likely) do not. They hire lobbyists, you do not. They win, congress wins, and you and I continue to struggle for good health.

Our government's influence over your nutrition is most powerful within the U.S. Department of Agriculture (USDA) and nowhere is the conflict involved with serving two masters greater. The USDA's mission is to encourage new markets and job opportunities within agriculture and food production while at the same time making recommendations and policy regarding what Americans should eat. Even within their mission the conflict is evident. The priority in food and nutrition policy is to encourage jobs and economic development first, and provide nutrition information and guidelines second. So, on one hand they want to keep meat and dairy producers and farmers gainfully employed, and on the other hand they tell the public what they should be eating: jobs first, public health second, or as I like to put it win, win, lose. Everything that comes out of the offices of the USDA and the Centers for Disease Control must first be carefully reviewed so that it does not damage the food industry. Remember, it's jobs first, public health second.

Aldana On The Hill

A few years ago I was invited to Washington to meet with the Secretary of Health and Human Services. In that meeting, we had the Secretary, and directors of Medicare, Medicaid, the FDA and USDA. I was summoned to Washington to give my opinion on what these organizations could do to improve public health. I mentioned this conflict and how it has created much of our unhealthy food culture. I suggested that the nation's best health experts at the National Institutes of Health be given the task of making nutrition recommendations to the public. They have no conflict of interest; their only mission is to improve the health of all Americans. That meant that the USDA could focus on what it does best—promoting jobs and markets in agribusiness. The response from the director of the USDA was swift and immediate, "That will never happen." Perhaps as one with extensive government experience he was simply stating the fact that any change to the current system would be impossible.

This was one of several recommendations I made to the group and I appreciated the opportunity I had to share my thoughts. Upon reflection, my eyes had once again been opened to the realities of federal government. Once ideologies and agencies are put into place change is almost impossible. A year or two later, I was in another professional meeting where we were discussing nutrition recommendations for the prevention and treatment of diabetes. Diabetes experts from within the CDC were expressing their frustrations regarding the same conflict I'd seen in Washington earlier. They were making recommendations about nutrition and lifestyle change for those with type II diabetes, but by the time the recommendations made it to the public they had been altered in such a way that they would not jeopardize anyone's job or any single industry. Their hands had been tied by the priority to maintain jobs and the economy first, above public health. For example, a recommendation to eat less sugar is a very good idea for those with type II diabetes, but it would hurt those in the sugar industry and so it was removed from the recommendations. Altering and changing recommendations in an effort to support the food industry is business as usual within our federal government.

I no longer care to meet with congressional committees or participate in federal panels; it's just too frustrating for me. My decision to no longer participate was made just a few years ago when I was working with Senator Orrin Hatch, a ranking member of the Senate Committee on Finance. I wanted the Senator's support for the Health Promotion First Act of 2007. He was very familiar with this bill and I asked if he would support it. I should not have been disappointed by his response, but I was. He said, "I cannot give you my support for this bill until I see how much support there is in the committee." In other words, the ranking member of the Senate Committee on Finance was more interested in the Democrat/Republican political battle than the health issues of American citizens. To his credit, he has been serving in the Senate for decades, so he clearly understands politics, but I wonder if his desires to maintain political power have clouded his view of the world we all live in. To maintain my own sanity, I'm better off not being involved with the federal government.

Frustrations With The Fed

While you and I are trying to have good health and a high quality life, our federal government is funding efforts that are working against us. In 1995, the USDA created Dairy Management, Inc., a nonprofit organization charged with increasing dairy consumption in the United States.[3] You have probably heard that Domino's pizza now sells Domino's American Legends pizzas, Pizza Hut has Cheesy Bites pizza, Wendy's has a new "Double Melt" sandwich and Burger King offers a Cheesy Angus Bacon. What you may not know is how these new products came to be. With taxpayer funding, Dairy Management has been working with the fast food industry to create products that contain more cheese. So while the USDA is making recommendations that you and I cut back on the amount of saturated fat we consume every day they are also funding one of the largest increases in cheese consumption in modern history. In a report to congress, Dairy Management stated that with their marketing efforts dairy farmers are now selling nearly 30 million more pounds of cheese. Fast food restaurants are selling more cheese-rich foods than ever. Of course, the fast food industry will claim they are just "offering consumers what they want, where and when they want it."

There are departments within the USDA devoted to marketing beef, pork, potatoes and other products. Dairy Management is the largest of all these departments with annual expenditures of $136 million. They also received $5.3 million from the Agriculture Department to promote dairy sales overseas while at the same time the department's Center for Nutrition Policy and Promotion spent $6.5 million promoting healthy diets. So, on one hand our federal government is encouraging us to eat a healthy diet, while on the other hand it is funding and supporting consumption of the very foods we should be avoiding.

The aggressive marketing tactics of the dairy industry don't end with cheese. Everyone knows the "Got milk?" slogan. Perhaps you have seen commercials on TV promoting the benefits of milk as an effective weight loss strategy. In an effort to support dairy farmers, the USDA and the dairy industry spent hundreds of millions of dollars promoting the supposed weight loss benefits of dairy. This benefit is a myth. A recent review of the studies that have looked at the ability of dairy products to aid in weight loss tells a very different story.[4] There have been 49 different studies that have looked at whether or not a diet that includes dairy foods can contribute to weight loss. Of these 49 studies, 41 failed to show any connection at all between dairy foods and weight loss. Three of the studies actually reported that people who ate dairy foods gained weight. The remaining five studies suggested that dairy products could contribute to weight loss. Not surprisingly, three of the five studies that showed positive weight loss effects were funded by the dairy industry. All told, research shows that dairy products have little, if any, effect on weight control—but that's not the story you've heard. Millions were spent convincing you that if you eat lots of dairy, you'll lose weight. From a business perspective, those millions of dollars was money well spent because people bought the message hook, line and sinker as milk sales soared. This is just one more example of how our desires for good health are being thwarted by an unhealthy food culture created by the very government agencies that should be protecting us.

You've Been Duped

Up to this point, we have discussed how you have been manipulated by the food industry, federal government and conflicted nutrition professionals. To help you understand how this actually affects your daily food choices, let's do some role-playing. Pretend you are the marketing director at a large food corporation, like Mars Incorporated, which is the candy company that makes Snicker's, Milky Way, Twix, Skittles and M&M's. Everyone knows that the candies you make are delicious, sugary treats that possess few health-promoting qualities. Your challenge is to sell as much candy as you can so you can meet your quarterly sales goals and keep your shareholders and investors happy. Remember, the foods you produce are not considered healthy, but you must still convince consumers to buy lots of your foods.

If you think like a marketing professional, you can probably create some effective selling tactics. Here are a few I came up with:

- Make things look complicated so that consumers will see this complexity and assume it must be okay or at least not question anything you say.
- Highlight any healthy aspects of your foods and never mention the bad parts.
- Understand that most consumers can be easily tricked with color and health messages.
- Get the blessing of the nutrition priesthood to validate what you are doing.
- Convince consumers that obesity is caused by lack of physical activity, not unhealthy food.

Let's see how these tactics actually work. You are likely familiar with the nutrition labels on all foods sold in the United States. The standard nutrition label that appears on our foods is one of the outcomes of years of conflicted government, industry and nutrition priesthood efforts. I included one here so you can see how it works.

Nutrition Information For A Snicker's Bar

Nutrition Facts

Serving Size 1 (2 oz) (57.0 g)

Amount Per Serving	
Calories 280	Calories from Fat 130
	% Daily Value *
Total 14g	**21%**
Saturated Fat 5g	**26%**
Trans Fat 0g	
Polyunsaturated Fat 3g	
Monounsaturated Fat 6g	
Cholesterol 5mg	**2%**
Sodium 140mg	**6%**
Total Carbohydrate 35g	**12%**
Dietary Fiber 1g	**5%**
Sugars 30g	
Protein 4g	
Vitamin A 0%	Vitamin C 0%
Calcium 4%	Iron 2%

*Percent Daily Values are based on a 2,000 calorie diet.

This is the nutrition label for a Snicker's bar, which is one of the products sold by the Mars company. It is also one of the products that uses marketing techniques and tactics to get you to buy more. Do you know what percent daily value means? How about international units? Are you really interested in how much vitamin C there is in your Snicker's bar? How about polyunsaturated fat and monounsaturated fat grams? Does anybody even look at this let alone understand it?

About half of all adults look at nutrition labels the first time they purchase a product and most of them are looking at the number of calories listed.[5] The labels are being viewed by some, but in general most of the information on these labels is completely ignored by the public. Unless you have an in-depth understanding of human nutrition, the information contained on these labels does little to help you make healthy nutrition choices. Just because people look at the labels doesn't necessarily mean that they make healthy choices. The complexity of the labels is exactly what the food industry wants. In fact, the food industry was involved in developing the labels. These labels don't really tell you what you should and shouldn't eat. Rather, they show you grams and percentages. You are left to do the calculations and determine if the food is part of a healthy lifestyle. The food industry loves these labels because they have little, if any, impact on your purchasing decisions. It's yet another win, win, lose scenario. The government can state it has produced food labels the public can use, the food industry still maintains high sales due to the complexity of the labels, and you, the consumer, are still likely to continue buying unhealthy foods that lead to chronic disease.

Remember, your job as the marketing director at Mars is to sell food. The food labels don't hurt your sales, but they don't help either. What would really be helpful is if you could highlight the few good nutrition elements that your foods contain. So, you label any "healthy" elements in green (because green means go) and you place it on the front of the package. If you look at a Snicker's bar, you'll see a label that looks just like the one below with one exception. The label shown here is in black and white, and the one on the front of your Snicker's bar is bright green. Remember, green means go. This new label was solely developed by the food industry. It's called the "facts up front" label. Always pursuing better sales, the food industry has developed these self-serving facts up front labels to expose every customer to the nutritional "benefits" of eating a Snicker's bar. By making them green, and including only the nutrition facts that aren't so bad, Mars is selling a Snicker's bar as something it's not: a healthy part of your diet.

CALORIES	TOTAL FAT	SAT FAT	SUGAR	SODIUM
280	**14g**	**5g**	**30g**	**140mg**
14% DV	22% DV	25% DV	*	6% DV

You'll be seeing a lot more of these because the government is currently setting rules and regulations on a similar looking label. I consider it just one more set of conflicted government guidelines designed to promote jobs and industry first and public heath second.

Another labeling trick that helps sell more food involves hiding the not-so-healthy ingredients. Because sugar comes in different forms, food producers often use different names for sweeteners. Take a look at one of your favorite foods and you might see words like invert sugar, fruit juice concentrates, corn sweetener, corn syrup, molasses, cane juice, cane syrup or agave, among many others. Then, there are the "ose" sugars, like dextrose, fructose, glucose and fructose. Because total sugar content may be divided among many different sweeteners, those ingredients may appear farther down the list, giving the appearance that the food you're eating does not contain much sugar when in fact it does. By using different sweeteners, food producers can avoid the word sugar, which might scare you away and decrease sales.

The U.S. Congress recently passed a law requiring restaurants to also provide these same nutrition labels on their foods. In theory, this may be a pretty good idea, but studies on the impact of labeling have painted a different picture. A review of all the studies that have looked at the impact of restaurant nutrition labels shows that some people might look at the labels, but they are still not making healthier choices or decreasing the number of calories consumed.[6–7] Other nutrition scientists have reported that these labels are not changing behaviors and the labels by themselves are not going to improve public health.[8]

The current requirements for nutrition labeling are a perfect example of what happens when several conflicted groups get together to solve a problem. We end up with a confused public that feels they cannot trust the food manufacturers or the federal government to watch out for their best interests. A survey by the FDA shows that 59% of Americans do not trust the food labels.[5] Fool me once, shame on you. Fool me twice, shame on me. The food industry has been fooling us for years and they have been doing so with the support of nutrition professionals and the federal government. No wonder most Americans no longer trust the food labels. I see nothing in the future that suggests that the food industry will stop their aggressive, self-serving activities.

In Europe, the food labeling system is different. The scientific community is in charge of making nutrition recommendations, and even though they still have to fight against the influences of the food industry, they appear more interested in public health than corporate profits. When you buy food in Europe the nutrition label on the front is color-coded red, yellow and green—the colors of a traffic light. Everybody understands red, yellow and green. Green means go, yellow means caution and red means stop. It's simple, people understand it and it helps them make healthy food choices. The European food industry unsuccessfully spent $1.5 billion lobbying against the European Union's approach. They aggressively fought any attempt at using a red light to suggest that any food was unhealthy, but eventually lost.[9] In Europe, nutrition recommendations are based on improving public health while in the United States recommendations are based on promoting jobs and profits. In the U.S., nutrition officials are influenced by food industries who say, "We believe the most effective programs are those that trust consumers and not ones that tell consumers what they should and should not eat." In other words, consumers should trust the food industry to look out for their best interests.

Self-Regulation Is No Regulation

Many politicians and nutritionists believe that if you leave the food industry alone they will do the right thing. They suggest that self-regulation is the best way to encourage the food industry to promote healthy foods. This philosophy suggests that those who profit from the foods we eat will consistently put public health before corporate self-interests. They point to the fishing and forestry industries as examples of how self-regulation can protect the environment and still keep companies profitable. Self-regulation works when an industry has a finite resource like fish and trees because if you fail to self-regulate and overfish or over harvest, the resource and the businesses that harvest them disappear. Self-preservation is a very good reason for self-regulation. Outside of these industries, if you plan on companies doing the socially responsible thing your plans will fail. All we have to do is look at the tobacco, alcohol and banking industries to see that self-regulation is no regulation. And no regulation equates to free reign to do whatever you need to do to make as much money as you can.[10] Public health does not have a chance of thriving in a corporate environment of self-regulation.

When threatened by possible government regulation, industries go on the offensive by re-asserting their commitment to public welfare and moral virtues. When they get caught, they hire PR firms to make the public like them again. The food industry has made multiple pledges to stop marketing to children, sell fewer unhealthy products in schools and label foods in responsible ways. Based on past experience, any promises of self-regulation by the food industry should be viewed with a high degree of skepticism.

But Wait, There's More

The food industry knows that you are more likely to buy foods that have nutrition information on the front of the package. To be sure, the nutrition labels, health claims and nutritional benefits really get consumers' attention. Wanting to sell more food, the food industry started using special terms like "less fat" "less sodium" "reduced fat" and "fat free" as well as health claims like "reduces cholesterol" and "reduces blood glucose." It's the wild wild west right now as the food industry ramps up their marketing efforts by promising consumers an endless array of health benefits associated with consuming their food products. And as the supplement industry and the food industry continue to merge, health claims have become food marketers secret sauce. Label any food product with a claim to improve health and sales will improve. Every once in a while a food producer will be slapped by a fine for making unsubstantiated claims, but in reality it's all just a game where the food producers are a few steps ahead of federal regulators. Just when the FDA shuts down one food health claim, another pops up in an endless game of "whack a mole." New regulations are written, lawyers are hired and loopholes are quickly exploited. Few industries are better at manipulating, influencing and sidestepping regulations designed to protect the public.

Real And Imagined Endorsements

Another tactic the food industry uses to influence consumer purchasing decisions is the use of real and imagined endorsements. Take a look at a box of Cocoa Puffs Cereal. Look on the side panel and you'll see the heart shaped label of the American Heart Association (AHA). This American Heart Association label means that the food manufacturer has met some sort of nutrition recommendation set by the AHA. It also means that the food manufacturer has given the AHA thousands of dollars. In essence, the food producers have purchased the blessing of the AHA. The food producers will sell more of their product with the official blessing of the AHA and the AHA makes millions of dollars each year in labeling fees. Cocoa Puffs wins, the AHA wins, and you get to eat Cocoa Puffs without knowing that you have been duped into thinking you are doing something healthy. I know many of you are disappointed that Cocoa Puffs are not part of a healthy breakfast, but they're not. Food producers use the endorsements of health authorities like the AHA, sports figures, professional organizations and any other famous person who can influence your decision to purchase.

One of the sneakiest endorsements is really not an endorsement at all. The other day my son brought home a package of watermelon-flavored Sour Patch soft and chewy candies. These candies are your typical sweet and sour candy snacks. It has no redeeming health qualities whatsoever, but it is fun to eat. It's just a bag of sugar and yet when I turn the bag over I see an "endorsement" from the federal government. On the back of the bag is this label: "To be enjoyed as part of a healthy, active lifestyle. To learn more about nutrition, visit **www.choosemyplate.gov**." To make you feel good about purchasing Sour Patch soft and chewy candy, the manufacturer has posted an unofficial endorsement by the U.S. government. It's not really an endorsement at all it's just a health message. But, having a health message on the package is an implied endorsement that will convince some people to purchase. Look at a box of Keebler graham crackers. On the back you'll see the nutrition pyramid from **www.choosemyplate.gov** and more health information from the USDA. Even though graham crackers are made of flour, sugar and fat, you might be convinced to buy them just because you see the nutrition pyramid on the back. They have 0 grams of trans fats, no cholesterol and are a good source of calcium…at least that's what the marketing team at Keebler wants you to know.

Many farmers and food producers have banded together to create their own industry groups such as the pork industry, the dairy industry and the wheat industry. The Whole Grain Council is a group of wheat growers and wheat producers that work together to increase wheat sales. They have come up with their own label called the Whole Grain Stamp. Any food producer that meets the rules and pays a fee of $1,000 to $10,000 per year gets the right to use the Whole Grain Stamp on their food package. Some foods that carry this stamp are actually healthy, but many are not. The rules for using this stamp are very loose and deceptive. But the impact of the stamp on increasing sales is impressive.

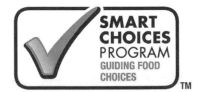

They know that as a consumer you will see a health label like the stamp and purchase more foods that have the stamp. Pepsico turned up its nose at all the other labels and started their own called Smart Spot. Over 250 Pepsico products now carry the Smart Spot label. By creating some arbitrary nutrition rules, certain foods can qualify to get the Smart Choices label, which creates an interesting scenario. If some of your foods have Smart Choices labels what does that say about all the other foods your company sells? They're "not so smart" choices? Some of the nation's biggest food producers like General Mills, Kellogg's and Kraft Foods have created their own self-serving labels while nutritionists look the other way.

The foods you see in grocery stores are now plastered with these self-serving labels and stamps. Each food producer is trying to beat the competition with bigger and bolder health claims and labels while you, the consumer, is left to figure out what you should or shouldn't eat. The food industry makes the rules that support their marketing efforts. Not surprisingly, lots of "good choice" labels end up on foods that do nothing to promote your good health. For a while you could find the smart labels on boxes of Froot Loops and Cocoa Krispies.

Deflecting Attention

If you go to the websites of many of the large food producers you will see materials, games and resources that have been developed to encourage physical activity. An effective way to deflect your attention from the fact that many foods are unhealthy is to refrain from the entire discussion. The food industry would like you to believe that the obesity and diabetes epidemic is not really about unhealthy foods, but simply a lack of physical activity. To solve the obesity and diabetes problem all you have to do is move around more, and here are some great games and resources to help you do just that. By diverting your attention to your lack of physical activity, the blame for poor health is transferred from unhealthy foods to sedentary lifestyles. That way the food industry can continue to aggressively market unhealthy foods while at the same time be seen as protectors of public health. By refocusing your attention on your lack of physical activity they are able to maintain the status quo and keep shareholders happy.

The Cavalry Is Not Coming

In moments of despair or trouble it is nice to call someone for help. Obesity, diabetes and chronic diseases have never been worse, and we are in trouble. Who can come to the rescue? Who is in a position to help us? This chapter has shown you that those who are in a position to help—our federal government and nutrition professionals—are conflicted. Their help is extremely limited despite their efforts. Those in a position to provide the most support for this problem are not now, nor in the near future going to be of much assistance. The cavalry is not coming, at least not for a long time. That means that you and I are alone in our efforts to improve our health. I wish it were otherwise, but your desires for good health run counter to those who are making money on the current culture they have helped create. Congress is unlikely to do anything to resolve these issues and you and I can blame them all we want for creating part of this culture, but nothing is going to change. I admit this is a very pessimistic view, but as I watch the obesity trends continue to rise and as I see people suffering from chronic diseases on a daily basis my hope for political and corporate solutions has faded.

I can only see one way out. The ONLY realistic solution to better health is for each of us to create our own culture of health. It is going to be up to you, your family, your employer and your church and community. Don't look for the food industry or the nutrition priesthood to ride to the rescue any time soon. If anything, they are to blame for getting us into this mess in the first place. Indeed, this is the only realistic solution I've seen actually work. The island natives that you've read about at the end of each chapter show us that this can be done without the cavalry. Their strategies combined with good scientific evidence show us that it is possible to create a healthy culture despite the conflicted political and cultural world in which we live. My pessimism pales in comparison to the optimism that I have for the future. Every day, all over the world, people like you and me are living healthy lives free from chronic diseases and obesity because we have learned to create and live in an alternative, healthier culture.

Island Native

I'm Sara Russell. I'm a 41-year-old mother of three and a stay-at-home mom living in South Bend, Indiana. About five years ago, I was feeling really in the dumps. I had gained about 20 pounds since high school and felt terrible about my health. I needed to do something to improve my self-image and my health. I was tired of who I had become and recognized that I needed an overhaul. I began by completely cutting out fast food and soda. I know the restaurants have nutrition information, but I never bothered to look at any of it. I just knew that a lot of the food I was eating was not healthy.

My biggest struggle was learning how to not overeat the wrong kinds of foods late at night. Rather than eat fast food, I started cooking, which allowed me to use more fruits and vegetables. If I did eat out with my children, I too would eat from the children's menu, which helped keep my serving sizes small. I started by making changes to my eating habits, but eventually realized that I also needed to be more active. I started walking every day and would push my youngest child in a stroller. After a while, my walk gradually turned into a slow, sustained jog. Between changes in my diet and activity level, I started to see some changes in both my health and my self-image. If I had one piece of advice for people trying to change I would say, "Don't get discouraged in the first two weeks. It will get better—I promise."

PART II

What To Do About It: How To Create A Better Culture

CHAPTER 8

Connecting The Dots

LET'S TAKE A MINUTE TO CONNECT THE DOTS BETWEEN OUR UNHEALTHY CULTURE AND YOUR ABILITY TO HAVE A LONG, HEALTHY LIFE. On a recent trip I was staying with some friends in Brooklyn, New York. As I walked around the neighborhood I tried to find a healthy place to eat. After walking about 10 blocks in each direction, I discovered a couple pizza places, a drugstore, Burger King, McDonald's and a convenience store. There were no grocery stores or delis. In this neighborhood, the majority of people walk and use public transportation to get around. If they want to grab a quick, healthy bite of food, it would require considerable time and travel to get it. Not all neighborhoods in Brooklyn are like this, but many are. Many neighborhoods across the U.S. are just like this. There are simply few options available to anyone who is striving to have a healthy diet. This is an example of the environmental influences that are a part of our culture and they have a direct impact on our health.

We don't typically think of our health in these terms, but where you live can influence your health. Where you work, where you go to school, your home environment, your community and neighborhood, and even church groups can have a large influence (good or bad) on your health. Those with higher incomes and higher levels of education can afford to live in areas where healthier foods are available and moreover, they can afford to purchase healthier foods. All of these factors are part of our culture and have a direct impact on our ability to live a healthy lifestyle. It is the most important piece of the good health puzzle and that is why it is the focus of this entire book. I like to think of it like a chemical reaction. To get a reaction started you have to add a catalyst, a substance that will get the whole reaction working. Our poor health is started by our unhealthy culture and environment; it's the catalyst that gets the whole thing started. The factors involved in our pathway to poor health have been identified. The pathway looks like this:

Culture → **Unhealthy Behaviors** → **Elevated Health Risks** → **Chronic Disease And Early Death**

It all starts when our culture and environment influences us to live our lives in a certain way. Either by habit, tradition or peer pressure, our culture has a tremendous influence on our behaviors. Our culture largely determines whether or not we exercise regularly, use tobacco or have a healthy diet. There are other behaviors that are influenced by our culture, including stressful living, poor sleep habits, poor driving habits, unsafe sex and drug abuse. All of these are important behaviors, but the majority of our chronic disease is being caused by just three: poor diet, lack of exercise and tobacco use. These unhealthy behaviors lead directly to elevated health risks such as high blood cholesterol, high blood pressure, high blood glucose and abdominal obesity. You'll remember from Chapter 1 that elevated health risks are the white smoke that warns us that something is wrong. These elevated health risks are nothing more than symptoms that the disease process is underway and with time, chronic disease and premature death are likely to occur. Culture, unhealthy behaviors, elevated health risks, chronic disease and early death (the dots) are all connected. Stated another way, how we decide to live our lives determines how and when we will die. Chronic disease and premature death are the outcome of poor lifestyle choices. The connection between each of these dots is not based on wishful thinking or personal testimonials, but decades of indisputable scientific evidence that continues to grow almost daily. This evidence proves that not only does our culture influence chronic disease and early death, but that changing this culture can prevent disease and improve quality of life.

Real Connections

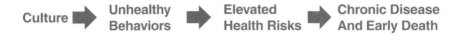

Let's take a look at how this works in the real world by talking about Mary. Mary lives in Brookfield, Illinois, a suburb of Chicago. Because Mary lives in the suburbs she must use a car as her primary method of transportation, which means she doesn't get very much physical activity by walking. Since most people who live in Brookfield commute to work every day they usually don't have much free time to cook meals. Of course, quick, convenient restaurants, especially fast food restaurants, are plentiful. Moreover, because of Mary's commute she doesn't have much free time to be regularly physically active. Most of her free time is devoted to her family and household duties—so the odds of her engaging in regular, vigorous physical activity are slim. Her busy work and family schedule combined with the location of her home have an impact on her behaviors, especially her nutrition and physical activity. This is just one example of how culture and environment can have a direct impact on health behaviors. Where people are born, grow up, live and work are the catalysts that influence how and when they will die.[1]

Even the state in which you live in can have a tremendous impact on your health. For example, in California, 12% of adults smoke, while in Arkansas it's double that at 24%. The gap is entirely due to differences in the culture and environment within each state. California has a culture that discourages tobacco use, while the culture in Arkansas is different. Culture has an influence on people in Brookfield, Illinois; it has an influence on people in California; it has an influence on the residents of Arkansas. What we eat, how much we eat, whether we use tobacco or whether or not we get regular exercise are influenced by our culture.

Despite the fact that she lives in the suburbs and doesn't get much exercise, Mary does have a healthy diet and she doesn't use tobacco. She is not overweight nor is she diabetic, but she does have high blood pressure, which increases her risk for cardiovascular disease. Is her high blood pressure caused by her behavior? Do unhealthy behaviors cause us to have elevated risk factors? These questions indeed open up the argument about genetics versus behavior (nature versus nurture). Do elevated health risks and chronic disease occur because of some uncontrollable influences such as genetics, random chance, or acts of God or are they actually the result of the daily choices we make about food, exercise and tobacco? Is poor health or good health for that matter, influenced by our personal behaviors or is it just the outcome of the lottery of life where health winners and losers are chosen entirely at random? The correct answer is both, but it's far from an even split.

If all our elevated health risks were caused by genes, all the healthy eating and exercise in the world would have little impact on lowering the risks. If it's caused by proteins we inherited from our parents, we have only our parents to blame and there is no need to spend any time reading this book. There are occasions when high blood pressure, cholesterol and glucose are caused by an inherited genetic mutation. But these are rare, occurring in less than 5% of the population. That means the remaining 95% of all elevated health risks are caused by our individual choices, **not our genetics**.

The pharmaceutical industry is very aware that only a slight number of high blood cholesterol cases are genetic. They would like you to think that most high blood cholesterol cases are genetic and that your only option is drug therapy. Of course, drug therapy is not the only option. Our unhealthy behaviors are the cause of almost all elevated health risks. This explains why so many Americans have so many elevated health risks. Our human genetic code has not changed in the last 30 years, yet the prevalence of elevated health risks has gone way up. We have drastically changed the amount of salt, sugar and fat we eat. The additional saturated fat is the primary reason we have high blood cholesterol. The extra fat and salt cause elevated blood pressure, and all the processed food we eat is a big contributor to elevated blood sugar and the subsequent development of diabetes. While our genes have remained unchanged, our culture has altered our health behaviors and has put us on the path to chronic disease.

What if you inherited a specific gene from your mother or father that increases your risk for cardiovascular disease? Such a gene does exist, it's called a chromosome 9p21 variant and if you have it, your chances of getting cardiovascular disease are higher than if you don't. But just because you have a genetic risk still doesn't mean you are destined to get the disease. One study looked at 8,000 individuals who have this gene. Even though they all have the gene those with a healthy diet have a much lower risk of heart attack than those with an unhealthy diet.[2] Those with the gene and a healthy diet did not have any increased risk for heart attacks. Even though they had a genetic predisposition to get heart disease, their risk was just as low as those without the gene. It appears that a healthy lifestyle can even help counteract the influence of some genes.

Win, Win, Lose With Paula Deen

Paula Deen is an American cooking show host from Savannah, Georgia. She has made a living teaching people how to cook delicious southern foods that are chock-full of salt, sugar and fat. She's published five cookbooks and is considered the queen of southern comfort food. She has a faithful group of followers who love to cook and eat foods that are a big part of the food culture in the deep south. For years she has been promoting the delicious benefits of southern cooking. Her cookbook aimed at children recommends cheesecake for breakfast and chocolate cake, French fries and meatloaf for lunch. What Paula hadn't been sharing with her followers is that after years of living this lifestyle she has become diabetic. She is a perfect example of how culture impacts behavior, risk and disease. Paula Deen, ever the business opportunist, is now a paid spokesperson for one of the largest diabetes treatment companies in the world called Novo Nordisk.[3] She has become wealthy promoting foods that lead to chronic disease and now she adds to her wealth by making money from the company that treats those same chronic diseases. The dots between culture and disease are connected and you get to be the loser in this win, win, lose scenario. Paula wins, Novo Nordisk wins, and you lose when you eat these foods, develop chronic disease, suffer and die prematurely.

If you are completely captured by our unhealthy culture you likely have a diet that includes a lot of processed foods, sugars, few fruits and vegetables or whole grains, and you don't move around very much. Actually, this sounds like a lot of people I know. With this type of lifestyle, it is common to have a waist circumference greater than 40 inches for men and greater than 35 inches for women. This type of lifestyle is also often accompanied with high blood triglycerides, high blood pressure, high blood glucose and low good cholesterol (HDL). If you have three or more of these risk factors you meet the definition of a person who has Metabolic Syndrome. This ominous sounding name simply means your body is currently developing several chronic diseases at the same time. Talk to any cardiologist and he or she will tell you they spend most of their time treating patients who have Metabolic Syndrome. If you have three or more of these risks you also have the need for intensive lifestyle modification.[4]

Here's the astonishing part: a recent national government survey showed that one out of three adults in the United States has it.[5] Here are some interesting facts about Metabolic Syndrome. You don't have to be overweight to have it (but it tends to be more common among those who have gained weight). It is more common among males than females and the older you become the more likely you are to get it. However, Metabolic Syndrome is not really related to gender or how old we are, it's actually determined by how much exposure we have to unhealthy behaviors.

Men typically have worse health behaviors than women, and the longer we live with poor health behaviors the more likely we are to get it. So, it's not really related to our age as much as how long we are exposed to unhealthy behaviors. If you are part of the 34% of adults in the United States with Metabolic Syndrome you are like a car that is not only blowing white smoke out of the tail pipe, but also leaking oil, antifreeze, power steering fluid and transmission fluid. The risk factors that you have are telling you that something is not right and that unless you do something to correct the problem, things are only going to get worse. The real problem is your unhealthy lifestyle.

It's pretty clear that almost all of our elevated health risks are caused by poor health behaviors, but what about the actual chronic diseases themselves? The major chronic diseases are pretty easy to identify because they are the leading causes of death in the U.S. Take heart disease for example. There are over 15 million adults in the U.S. currently suffering from heart disease. Of these 15 million cases of heart disease, it's estimated that around 82% are caused by poor lifestyle choices.[6] If you have friends or family members who have heart disease, there is an 82% chance that they developed the disease because of the unhealthy behaviors they adopted throughout their life. The other 18% of cases could be genetic or caused by environmental factors of which we have little control. Cancer is the second most common killer in the United States and it is estimated that 70% of all cancers are lifestyle related.[7] Additionally, 70% of all strokes and 91% of all type II diabetes can be explained by an unhealthy diet and lack of exercise.[8]

There is no debate that some chronic diseases and health risks can be genetically inherited from our parents. What most people fail to realize is that it is inaccurate to blame our genes for poor health that was caused by our poor lifestyle choices. It's easy to blame our genes because doing so provides an escape for us: "Surely, I could not have done this to myself. This must be something I inherited from my parents."

If our unhealthy culture influences us to make poor lifestyle choices, and our poor lifestyle choices lead to elevated health risks and chronic disease, then it is logical to assume that it also is the main cause of premature death. When we talk about premature death we simply mean death that occurs earlier than it should have. Most people have already avoided premature death by wearing seatbelts, taking antibiotics, getting immunized and even keeping food refrigerated. Death comes to all, but for those who are under the influence of our western culture it tends to come earlier. On average, people who have unhealthy lifestyles pass away 10 to 20 years earlier than they should.[9] I can hear the skeptics right now asking, "How do you know it is really a 10 to 20 year difference?"

Data Connects The Dots

Let's get back to Mary from Brookfield, Illinois. When she was 39 years old she was asked to participate in a long-term research study called a cohort study. She was one of over 7,000 women who joined the study in 1970.[10] The researchers showed up at her home drew some blood, gave her a physical and asked questions about her nutrition, physical activity and other health behaviors. With her contact and medical information in hand, the researchers disappeared. Every few years they showed up and gathered more medical information. For Mary and all the other women, this research study continued for 30 years. During that time, many of the women developed chronic diseases and many died of cardiovascular disease, diabetes and other causes. With 30 years of data, the researchers began asking a lot of really interesting questions. They first wanted to know if health risks and health behaviors were the cause of chronic diseases and early death. They were able to split the women into two groups. One group of women had good health behaviors and low health risks. This group had normal blood pressure, cholesterol and glucose and they did not smoke and were not obese. The other group included women who had one or more of these five risk factors (high blood pressure, glucose or cholesterol, overweight or tobacco users). Once they had been split into these two groups they looked at all the chronic diseases and deaths to see which group had more. Only 20% of the women were low risk in all five areas; all the other women had at least one risk factor and were put into the second group. After 30 years, the women with two or more risk factors were five to six times more likely to die of cardiovascular disease and other causes.[11] Cardiovascular disease and death were rare in the first group and this group also had a higher quality of life and substantially lower health care costs. They could walk more, had better mental health and had far fewer cases of other chronic diseases.[12-13] Through their participation, Mary and all the other women in this study showed us that poor health behaviors and elevated health risks are clearly connected with cardiovascular disease and death. With this study, the ability of a healthy lifestyle to improve and extend our lives was just starting to be better understood.

In the past 50 years there have been hundreds of studies just like this one that have looked at the connections between behavior, risk, disease and death. These studies have included all races and ages as well as men and women and the rich and poor. Studies have been completed on Mexicans, Japanese, Chinese, British, French, Indians, Russians and almost every other sizable nationality in the world. All of them have included thousands of participants with some studies including over 300,000 adults followed for decades. Most of them have looked at many of the same behaviors and risk factors. They almost all include some type of poor health behavior like physical inactivity, tobacco use, alcohol consumption, poor diet and inadequate sleep. These studies have also included health risks like abdominal obesity, excess body weight, and high blood cholesterol, blood pressure, and blood glucose. All of them are designed almost identically: gather a bunch of health and disease information from a lot of people, step back and let them live their lives. Then keep track of who develops chronic diseases or passes away, and go back and start connecting the dots.

Rather than bore you with all the academic details, I'm going to summarize these findings into just a few points:[9]

- A healthy lifestyle can lower the risk of heart attack and heart disease death by 70 to 89%.
- If you have a healthy lifestyle you could expect to live between 10 and 20 years longer than those who don't have a healthy lifestyle.[14–15]
- Blood pressure drops with a healthy diet, aerobic exercise and reduced amounts of alcohol and sodium.
- Blood cholesterol improves when you eat more fiber, less saturated fat and cholesterol, and lose weight and exercise.
- Diabetes can be prevented, arrested and in many cases reversed when you have a healthy lifestyle. Almost all type II diabetes cases are caused by unhealthy lifestyles.[16]
- When you stop smoking, increase your physical activity, reduce alcohol consumption and improve your diet, you cut your risk of heart disease death by 20 to 40%.
- Exercise for the treatment of depression is just as effective as medications, but with no side effects.
- A healthy lifestyle prevents chronic diseases at any age.
- Excess weight, poor diet, physical inactivity and smoking account for most of the major diseases of modern society, including heart disease, stroke, diabetes, osteoarthritis, osteoporosis, colorectal cancer, depression and kidney disease.

I think you get the point. A lot of really good research has been completed and the connections between our culture, behaviors and disease are pretty much cemented in stone. Sometimes I think of this research as if it were a crystal ball. If the studies' participants had poor health behaviors and elevated health risks, chances were pretty high that their future included chronic disease and premature death. Fortunately, unlike this research, your future is not set in stone. Scientists show us that if you can adopt healthy behaviors you can prevent undue suffering and have a high-quality, long life. Your health can be improved and enhanced, but it's not always easy to do. A simple visit to the grocery store is a prime example of the challenges and misconceptions you will encounter. For example, you can go to the grocery store and see that a box of Kellogg's Corn Pops is being promoted as an excellent source of fiber and should be an essential part of a healthy diet. Kellogg's is promoting a lie when they suggest that crispy, glazed, crunchy, sweet Corn Pops should be part of a healthy lifestyle. Health researchers tell us what we need to do to have a healthy, disease-free lifestyle, while our culture and the food industry tell us an entirely different story.

It's Hard To Change

Long before the British Empire started colonizing Australia the aboriginal peoples had been living there for thousands of years. They had been living a typical hunter/gatherer lifestyle, consuming fruits and vegetables and animals found in their natural state. They had hard lives, but they didn't suffer from the chronic diseases we have today. They had a diet and physical activity regimen that could be envied today. As the colonizers brought new technologies and western culture to that continent the native people gradually adopted western ways of living. And just like us, their diets and exercise habits changed. They became fat, they lost their high levels of fitness and many of them became diabetic. They used to be a very healthy population, but with the new culture their health declined dramatically. Now, efforts are being made to help them regain their health. Of course, it's extremely difficult to give up this convenient new culture.[17] A similar effort is being made across many of the Native American populations in the U.S., but again, with the lure of delicious, convenient and relatively inexpensive processed foods it's very hard to give this culture up. The Australian aborigines and some of the Native American populations have made some progress in restoring their native cultures, diets and lifestyles but it's an uphill battle.

Think of the billions of dollars (yes, billions) being spent on weight loss programs including books, weight loss camps, surgery, pills and weight loss programs to help us regain our health. We hear promises of permanent weight loss, guaranteed results and the end of overeating, but in the end, most of us fail to achieve long-term weight loss and good health. We might have some success initially, which I call passing acculturation. This is when we are able to create and live in a new culture for a short period of time. Eventually, most people who lose weight will see the weight return. Whether it's an Australian aborigine, a Native American or you, we all struggle trying to escape the unhealthy culture in which we all live. There are so many ways that we fail to sustain a healthy culture and healthy behaviors. Maybe we are truly addicted to the salt, sugar and fat in our foods and our failure is nothing more than a relapse. We get busy and have great demands on our time, which forces us to neglect exercise and consume convenience foods. Maybe we succumb to the pleadings from our children to buy sugary treats and desserts. Perhaps we experience a major event such as a divorce, or the loss of loved one which can sabotage all of our efforts to have a healthy lifestyle. Sometimes it feels like our efforts to have a healthy lifestyle are being hampered by friends and family members when they make fun of our efforts to be healthy.

I've shared some of the personal stories of those who I call Island Natives. These individuals have not only created islands of health and healthy cultures, but they've also been able to sustain those efforts. Most people who are trying to be healthy will succeed at creating an island of health, and they will spend some time there, but eventually they move back to the mainland where they are quickly assimilated back into the western culture. They experienced a successful short term cultural shift that was unsustainable in the long term.

Is Anyone Able To Maintain A Healthy Culture?

Off the coast of Italy in the center of the Mediterranean Ocean is the island of Sardinia. Among the million or so people who live there is a large concentration of centenarians—people who are at least 100 years old. Not long ago, researchers from Belgium carefully studied the Sardinians to try to figure out how they can live such healthy, long lives.[18] There were differences in the number of centenarians in different regions of the island, with the more mountainous regions having the most centenarians. They determined that the reason these people live such long, healthy lives consists of a variety of factors including a strong culture of social support, a diet that consists of healthy foods found in their natural forms, regular daily physical activity and really good genes. Because they live on an island, researchers found that they all share a very similar genetic makeup. It may be that there are so many centenarians in this area because they all share a really healthy set of genes that has not been diluted by the outsiders who may introduce a less healthy gene pool. Most researchers agree that they probably do have a genetic advantage that when combined with a very healthy diet and active lifestyle helps them live as long as they do. All the talk and media coverage of the benefits of a Mediterranean diet got started with the findings on the Sardinians.

Far from Sardinia is another smaller set of islands that also have an abnormally high number of centenarians. In the sea of China about halfway between Japan and Taiwan is the island of Okinawa. Here, there is a very high portion of the population that lives active, high-quality lives well into their 100s. While trying to figure out their secret to good health, researchers learned several interesting facts: the Okinawans have their own distinct genetic pool, (hmm, that sounds familiar) which makes sense when you live on an isolated island. Additionally, their isolation also requires them to eat locally grown foods and to be more physically active.[19] The Sardinians and the Okinawans are two examples of people who live in a culture that encourages healthy living and who live long, healthy lives. The natural question to ask is, "Is their good health due to their genetics or their behavior, or both?"[20] Both groups have gene pools that have been isolated and both groups, compared to Americans, have very healthy diets and lifestyles. They have two really good things going for them: exceptionally good genes and extremely healthy lifestyles. Now, if we only had a third group that had a really healthy lifestyle, but did not share the same genes we might really be able to answer this question. Luckily, we can answer this question —we just need to go to California to do it.

Several decades ago, researchers began doing careful studies of members of the Seventh-day Adventist church. Started in 1863, this Protestant Christian religion has always encouraged its members to live wholesome, healthy lives. Adventists are known for their "health message" that recommends vegetarianism and expects adherence to the kosher laws in Leviticus 11. The church discourages its members from the use of alcohol, tobacco or illegal drugs. They have a day of rest every week, and maintain a healthy, low-fat vegetarian diet that is rich in nuts and beans. It is estimated that 35% of Adventists practice vegetarianism. Dozens of scientific papers have been written about the health benefits associated with this way of living. Adventists in California live four to 10 years longer than the average Californian. They have better health behaviors, significantly lower health risks and a dramatically lower prevalence of chronic diseases.[21] Unlike the Sardinians and the Okinawans, these Seventh-day Adventists have not been living in an isolated geographic area. They live all over the U.S. and in various parts of the world. They share the same culture and environment that you and I live in. They live around fast food restaurants, they see the same food industry lies and they experience the same changes in food quantity and quality that you and I are faced with.

One researcher calls the Seventh-day Adventists' ability to abstain from our modern culture as "immunity from our unhealthy culture."[22] When he compared the obesity rates of Seventh-day Adventists to non-Seventh-day Adventists, he found a very big difference. While you and I and most other people in the world gained weight from 1986 to 2006, these Seventh-day Adventists did not. They also had much healthier diets and lifestyles during this time. There's a case where genetics cannot be used to explain good health and longer lives. The Adventists who were included in these studies came from different ethnic and racial backgrounds representing a diverse gene pool. They live in different geographical areas of the United States and the world, speak different languages and are exposed to our unhealthy western culture in a variety of different ways. And yet, somehow, they appeared in many ways to be immune to the effects of our unhealthy culture. On a personal note, I am not a vegetarian, but I support anyone who wants to avoid eating meat. I do eat meat but I do so sparingly. I think our ancient ancestors ate meat, at least wild game and fish and though the meat we eat today is not quite the same, I do not believe it is a big factor in our pursuits for long-term health. But highly processed meats like bacon, sausage, and hot dogs, are very far from being in their natural form and should be avoided.

So how do they do it? How do these individuals live in the same culture and environment that you and I live in and somehow avoid the chronic disease and early death that effect so many of us? One item that is probably not a factor is their genetics, since they all have very different genetic backgrounds. One item that is a factor is that they avoid tobacco and alcohol which, just like the Mormons, has also extended life and reduced chronic disease prevalence. Just the avoidance of tobacco would dramatically extend the life of these individuals. But there is more to their good health than the avoidance of alcohol and tobacco. They also share strong social bonds and networks with others who are there to provide emotional, physical and moral support when needed. They have enjoyed initial improvements in good health which resulted in weight loss that continued for years, rather than stopping six or 12 months after the start of the program.[23] They have succeeded at creating and living on islands of health not just for a few months but for decades.

Forcing Healthy Culture on Pigs

Whether for religious reasons or for health reasons, many Adventists have chosen to live healthy lifestyles despite pressures to do otherwise. What would happen if people were forced to eat a healthy diet? That doesn't seem like a very nice thing to do, however, what would happen if you forced people to eat healthy? I don't see this as something we would ever want to do with people, but it would be interesting to see what happens to health if it could be done to pigs. One group of researchers did this very thing with 24 piglets.[24] Half of them were given a diet of cereals like corn and grain with lots of carbohydrates. The other half were given a diet much like the Paleolithic diet we discussed earlier in the book. These piglets ate vegetables, fruits, some tubers (starch vegetables like carrots and potatoes) and a little meat. They tried hard to provide the piglets with a diet that was representative of what our ancient ancestors might have eaten. After 17 months, the two groups of pigs were evaluated. The pigs that were forced to eat the Paleolithic diet weighed 22% less and had almost half the amount of fat.

This is really good if you're trying to promote health, but not very good if you're trying to sell bacon. The pigs with a Paleolithic diet had lower blood pressure and had a better response to insulin, meaning they were less prone to getting diabetes. By studying identical pigs that had different diets it became very apparent that what we put in our mouths has a big impact on our health risks and chronic diseases. The problem is people aren't pigs. It is difficult to force people to eat a specific diet and it isn't ethical. What we have seen from the Adventists is that with the right tools, motivation and support, it is possible to create and live in a healthy culture.

Violent Culture Change

This is not the first time cultures have changed. They've been changing for all of human history; it's just that the changes we are experiencing now are extreme. We're going from a traditional healthy culture to one that is very unhealthy, and this change is something we have brought upon ourselves. But, not all cultural changes are self inflicted. In 1989 the collapse of the Soviet Union resulted in the loss of economic aid and precipitated a nationwide economic crisis in Cuba.[25] This led to food and fuel shortages that reduced per person daily energy intake from 2,899 calories a day to 1,863 calories a day, and increased the prevalence of regular physical activity by nearly 70%. The prevalence of obesity was cut in half (14 to 7%) and deaths due to diabetes were cut by 51%. Coronary heart disease was down by 35%, strokes decreased by 20% and death by all causes was down by 18%. This experience was far from a voluntary lifestyle change program, but it demonstrates how western cultures can create an economic environment in which excess food and sedentary living can have very unfortunate side effects. An economic downturn produced dramatic food shortages which resulted in dramatic improvements in public health. This was not a typical food famine; its roots were economic in nature not climate in nature. Please don't misunderstand me; the last thing I want is for dramatic upheaval in our current economic system, that's a terrible way to improve public health. But it does illustrate that part of our problem is the culture of excess that we have created and when that excess disappears people are forced to make better lifestyle choices.

In the history of humanity countries and populations have been conquered by invading marauders. Each time this has happened the culture of the attackers usually becomes the dominant way of living and with time, becomes the new culture of the conquered people. This is a form of forced acculturation as a different culture is forced upon people. As unpleasant as this sounds, it has been happening for millennia. Americans are guilty of doing this very thing. Just ask any Native American population how much their culture has changed since the American colonizers showed up. This is the worst way to change the culture. There is an easier way to do it.

Proof This Works

Let me give you a realistic example of how people solve this problem right now. A few years ago, I was asked to be a team leader on a really large study that was going to look at the impact of a healthy lifestyle on risk and chronic disease. We recruited a group of 365 middle-aged working adults to participate in a lifestyle change program designed to help them eat a healthier diet and get regular physical activity. Each of these individuals participated in an intensive six-week program with information much like what you are learning in this book. Over the course of 18 months, we gathered data on physical activity, nutrition and health risks.[26–28] The participants learned about the importance of healthy lifestyles, and they gained and improved their motivation. They also had the chance to practice different skills and strategies needed to adopt healthy behaviors, and they learned how to change their own environment to make healthy behaviors easier. The adults in the study were typical, middle-aged working adults who wanted help improving their health. They were somewhat motivated to be there and they had to pay $280 for the opportunity. Motivation is one of the critical pieces to creating a healthy culture. Those who participated in the behavior change program were matched with individuals just like them who were not participating in anything. This was our control group.

Here is what we found: Six weeks after the program began, everyone had increased their physical activity level by at least 30% and improved their nutrition. In just six weeks, the entire group of program participants showed significant improvements in their blood pressure, cholesterol and blood glucose (a predictor of diabetes). On top of that, they all lost weight. These are pretty dramatic changes in just six weeks and we were pleased to have such an effect.

But ever the skeptic, I wanted see if there were any long-term behavior changes. So, we analyzed all the data again after two years had passed, and sure enough they had maintained their healthy behaviors for at least two years. Health risks were dramatically lower from where they started and they were well on their way to preventing, arresting and reversing many chronic diseases. These were real people with real jobs working in various cities in the central United States who had been inundated with our unhealthy western culture. This program proved that with the right approach, people can do more than have temporary successes; they can create and live on an island of health that improves their health, lengthens their life and improves their quality of life. These studies show us how we win the battle for better health.

There are three simple steps to making this work. The rest of this book is devoted to helping you find success with each of these three steps. And like the participants in the studies I've published, when these steps are completed, good things will start happening to your health.

Island Native

My name is Michael Petit. I'm a supervisor at a manufacturing plant in Milwaukee, Wisconsin. My employer decided to pay for all employees to get their blood screened. I guess the boss is trying to keep us healthy. I found out that I was type II diabetic and I had no idea. I'm a pretty big guy, but I never considered myself to be obese. With a BMI of 34, it turns out I was. With the knowledge that I was type II diabetic and obese I guess I got a little scared.

Thirty-four other employees and I who were diabetic were invited to participate in a lifestyle change program offered by my employer. With the help of our on-site safety nurse, and an intern from the local university we began weekly classes, exercise sessions and team competitions to help us change our lifestyles. I learned how my lifestyle was connected to my health risks, I got more motivated, and we learned new skills like how to shop for healthy foods, cooking and how to exercise. I also got to participate in team sports with other employees. It was actually kind of fun to work with others. We were permitted to exercise three times a week while at work. With the changes in my nutrition and physical activity, it didn't take long for me to see really big changes in my health risks. After two years of starting this program, I am still diabetes free. I've learned new ways to live my life. To be honest with you, this experience has changed my life. I started dating someone, I moved out of my mother's house, I'm proud of myself and I like myself. I have no intentions of ever going back to my old ways of living.

If I could say one thing to people who were thinking about doing this I would say don't get discouraged when you have some setbacks. Stop, think what you're doing, and get back on your island.

CHAPTER 9

Step 1—Find A Reason To Change

OUR UNHEALTHY CULTURE IMPACTS OUR HEALTH BECAUSE IT HAS A DIRECT IMPACT ON OUR BEHAVIORS. JUST ABOUT ANYTHING WE DO IS A BEHAVIOR, AND SOMETIMES THESE BEHAVIORS LEAD TO GOOD HEALTH AND SOMETIMES THEY ARE DETRIMENTAL TO IT. Smoking, not wearing a seatbelt, eating unhealthy foods, lack of regular exercise, working in a high stress environment, consuming too much alcohol and not taking prescribed medications are examples of unhealthy behaviors.

Getting healthy is all about adopting and maintaining behaviors that promote health. It doesn't do much good to adopt a healthy behavior for a short amount of time only to later abandon it. When the behavior stops, the health benefits that are associated with it will also end. Most people can easily try a new behavior, at least for a while. Just take a look at people who have been successful at quitting smoking. The average ex-smoker will quit (short term adoption) at least four times before they are successful at becoming completely tobacco free.[1] To be sure, real health benefits come to those who can acquire new health behaviors and keep those behaviors for the rest of their lives.

There are some very elaborate theories and explanations about how people change behaviors. There are hundreds of books and thousands of research articles on this process. All of this information is helping us figure out the best way to help people change behaviors. Unfortunately, most of it is written in academic language that I like to call psycho/social mumbo-jumbo. Scientists and academics understand it all very well but the average person, who perhaps needs behavior change help the most, won't understand much out of this research. My business partner Dr. Troy Adams and I have been successful using this behavior change science, but we've had to boil it down to its most important elements.[2] We like to call it the secret sauce of behavior change. But, it's not really secret and it's actually more of a process than a sauce. The truth is people get more excited when we talk about the secret sauce than when we talk about evidence-based, behavior modification paradigms.

This secret sauce provides an easy-to-follow process that can be used to change any behavior. We've been using this process with almost one million people in the U.S. There are three steps you must follow in order to be successful in changing behaviors.

1. **Find a reason to change**
2. **Learn new skills**
3. **Get help from others**

These steps may not look like much on the surface, but there is a lot of vital information packed into each step. Changing behaviors is probably one of the hardest things that humans can do. Despite our best intentions most of us fail at changing behaviors. Remember, smokers fail four times on average before they successfully quit. Human behavior is a complex interaction between our bodies, brains and environment. We have to rely on our senses to figure out what's going on around us and adapt. Behavior is literally nothing more than our reactions to our surroundings. Some aspects of our behaviors are emotional, physical, mental and even spiritual. This complexity is one reason so much research and investigation has been done to figure out how we change. Fortunately, the three steps we're going to talk about provide some simple guidelines that make a really complicated process easier to do. The steps will help you as you make changes in your health behaviors, but as you are about to see, you are already doing the three steps—you just don't know it. Let me give you an example.

My family and I have a good friend who recently turned 80. He has been obese all of his adult life. Fortunately for us, we still have him around even though most people who are obese rarely live past 65. Six months before his 80th birthday, we spoke and he told us of his plans to lose weight. He said, "The next time you see me I'm going to be 80 pounds lighter for my 80th birthday." Sure enough at his birthday party he announced that he had lost 80 pounds.

We hardly recognized him. When visiting with him about his accomplishment I asked him why, after all these years, did he suddenly decide to change his behaviors and lose weight? He had previously had both knees replaced and for many years had been suffering from a variety of obesity-related conditions. He replied, “I’m getting older and I think it’s time I paid more attention to my health.” For some reason he felt compelled to get serious about his health after having neglected it for most of his life. Step one of the behavior change secret sauce is to find a reason to change. For him, that reason was because he could see how his unhealthy behaviors were having a large impact on his health and after 50 years this reason became important enough for him to do something about it. It’s as if he reached a motivational tipping point where his desires to change were able to overcome any and all resistance to change.

Everyone always asks how he lost the weight. That’s where step two came in. He needed to learn new skills and strategies that were going to help him get rid of the extra weight. Working with his physician, he put himself on a very strict low-carb diet. He consumed a lot of vegetables and lean cuts of meat and very few carbohydrates. More importantly, he dramatically reduced the number of calories he was eating throughout the day. In addition to his dietary changes, he began doing water aerobics every day at the local community pool. Weight loss at its core is really all about calories-in versus calories-out. Consuming fewer calories and expending more through physical activity is the only way anyone can actually lose weight. The skills that he needed to be successful included learning how to prepare, cook and eat foods that were low in calories. He also learned how to rearrange his schedule so that he could spend time every single day working out at the pool. He also learned how to shop for and purchase foods that were part of his new diet. Lastly, he admits that he had help from others, which is what step three is all about. He had help from his doctor, but more importantly he had support from his spouse who was diligent in joining him for water aerobics every single day. Every single day the two of them went to the city pool to exercise. Of course, help from others isn’t just limited to actual people. Help from others can also refer to rules, policies and changes in our environment that make it easier for us to be successful. Our family friend established a few rules to guide his actions, which included not eating after 7:00 p.m., limiting sweets and desserts to once a week and getting an hour of exercise every day.

At the time he didn’t know anything about the behavior change secret sauce, he was just doing what he thought was best. In hindsight however, it’s easy to see that there was actually some order to his process. That order is nothing more than the three simple steps which comprise the secret sauce. After being immersed in an unhealthy western culture for most of his life, this friend was able to successfully alter his behaviors and create an alternate culture for himself, one that included healthy nutrition and regular physical activity. We are all so happy for him and his success, but I can't stop thinking about why it took him so long to get serious about it. You would think that after two knee replacement surgeries, decades of poor health and a poor quality of life that he would have been sufficiently motivated to do something about it sooner. But motivation doesn't always work that way. It's far more complicated. Something about the thought of reaching the age of 80 and being obese did not sit well with him, so he decided to act. He finally had a sufficient reason to change.

You too have used all three behavior change steps as you have picked up new behaviors in your life. Think about one of your behaviors. It can be anything, such as brushing your teeth, cleaning your room, eating whole-grain bread, not smoking, being kind to others, etc. Think about this one behavior and let me ask you a few questions. Why did you do it? You might have to think hard, but there is a reason. Maybe it's a habit you have created, but even that habit started because there was something you wanted. The behavior I picked was growing a garden. I grow a garden every year. I grow this garden because I like the taste of the fruits and vegetables that I grow. I also like to be outside in the fresh air working the soil. My reasons for growing a garden are strong enough to overcome any resistance I have towards not growing a garden. I understand what it takes to grow garden, I've learned about gardening, and over time I picked up a few new skills, knowledge and tools that I need to be successful. On a regular basis I get an e-mail from my local county extension office that contains great tips and gardening "how to" articles. I also know that my family loves to eat the produce that I grow and the joy I get in seeing the satisfaction on their faces makes me want to do it again next year. They give me support and encouragement. So here we have an example of a simple behavior where each of the three steps is used to help make the behavior permanent. I had a good reason to change. I acquired some new skills and tools to help me stick to it and I rely on the help and support I get from others. I use the behavior change secret sauce in my own life. If you look carefully at your own behaviors you will see that you have been following the same three simple steps. The challenge for each of us is to learn how to use these three steps going forward as we battle for healthier behaviors.

Failure Is Part Of The Process

The first time you rode a bicycle you probably lost your balance and fell to the ground. Your sense of balance and coordination had to adjust to the unique demands of riding a two-wheeled machine. Everyone fails to ride a bike in the beginning, but with each failure we get a little better and a little better until after a while we alter our actions enough to be successful. The same thing happens when we start a new behavior; failure is actually part of the process. After spending my whole life studying how to get people to have healthy lifestyles there is one main message that I keep finding: Adopting and maintaining new behaviors is very hard to do and most will fail the first time. New behaviors are exactly that—new. They require us to learn new ways of thinking and living. They require us to step out of our comfort zone and try something new and unfamiliar. They require change and for many people change is very hard to do. This is one reason why my friend maintained his obese lifestyle for 50 years. He wasn't interested in changing until it was apparent that his health was in jeopardy.

We don't like to fail. We want to be successful and we want to be successful the first time. Unfortunately, that is not how we change behaviors. The actual process of failing gives us the strength and motivation we really need to succeed. In some ways it's impossible to succeed without failing first. When we understand that failure is actually a natural and important part of the process, the first thing we probably ought to do is stop calling it a failure. It is more like fine-tuning our efforts or slowly building upon our previous experiences until we finally get it right. So long as we're moving in the right direction, our efforts to be healthy will be rewarded. In my mind I can imagine former smokers getting frustrated and upset with every failed attempt to quit not knowing that failing is actually part of the process. Believe it or not, every time you fail to maintain a healthy behavior you are that much closer to making it a permanent part of your life. This is because our desire to change behaviors is influenced by how ready we are.

A utility company that I work with has 4,000 employees who are trying to adopt healthy behaviors. We studied these employees quite extensively and in many ways they're just like the rest of us. I can place every one of them into one of four readiness categories. These categories correspond to how ready a person is to make lifestyle changes. One thousand of these employees or about 25% already have the healthy behaviors they need for a long, healthy life. They've already changed behaviors. All they really need to do now is maintain. Another 25% of these employees are thinking about making behavior changes—they like the idea, and with a little education and encouragement they are going to be successful. This group is ready to make changes, all they need is a little help, a little encouragement and for someone to show them the way. Then there's the next 25% of employees, another 1,000 people who aren't quite as ready. They are going to need lots of coaxing and maybe even a few subtle threats and bribes. They understand they should be making a change, they understand the risks to their health and their quality of life, but they're just not quite ready for action. We can offer them rewards if they make changes or maybe even make them pay more for health insurance if they don't, but in general they're going to need some pretty serious persuasion before they are going to get serious about adopting new behaviors.

Everyone knows someone who is in this last category. It's the remaining 25% of people at this company. They are going to change behaviors when pigs learn to fly or hell freezes over, whichever one happens first. They have little interest in changing health behaviors. They may think that since they feel fine there's no reason to change behaviors. Typically they are the young (younger than 35) who think that they are somehow immortal or unaffected by health risks or unhealthy behaviors. To some degree they are correct. It's possible to have a very unhealthy lifestyle and even have elevated health risks and not experience the onset of major chronic disease for several decades. They are probably carrying around an extra 20 to 50 pounds of weight. They have no interest in adopting and maintaining healthy lifestyles right now because they believe the statement my father taught me, "If it ain't broke, don't fix it." They feel fine, they have no pain and their lives are too busy to worry about health—they have no reason to change. Since step one of the behavior change process is to have a reason, it is unlikely they will succeed at changing behaviors.

The Four Categories Of Change Readiness

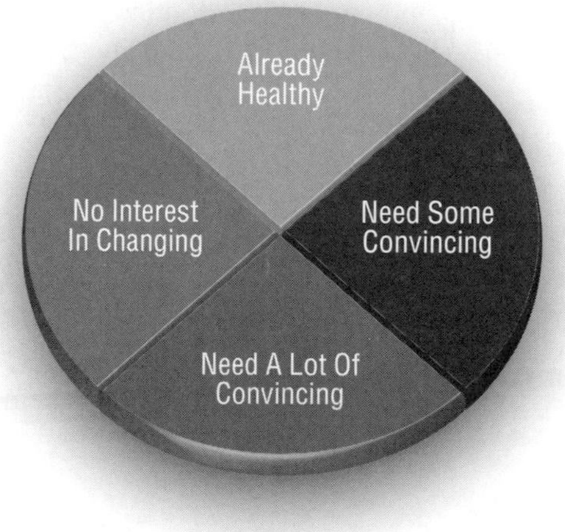

All of us fit into one of these four categories. Depending on the health behavior, it is possible to be in more than one category at the same time. For example, if you are a non-smoker, you are already doing the healthy behavior of avoiding tobacco. Since your behavior is a healthy one, you have no reason to change. But maybe you don't exercise regularly and you don't have much desire to start exercising. If you don't have a good reason to start exercising, all the exercise tools, strategies and support from others probably won't help you become physically active. You're not ready or at least you don't have a really good reason to change. As we carefully work through each of the three steps for success, we're actually working our way through each of these four readiness categories until we reach the point where we can maintain new behaviors for life. These categories help me remember that not everybody is ready or willing to change behaviors. Despite all of the tremendous benefits that come from having a healthy lifestyle, people won't adopt healthy behaviors until they're fully ready. With the passage of time, our values and motivations will change. Anyone who isn't ready for change now may be ready to change later, even if it's 80 years later.

Accurate Knowledge Gives You Power To Change

You wouldn't be reading this book if you didn't have at least some interest in changing your lifestyle. You probably have thought about how your life would be better if you lived differently. Thinking about it is a good start, but what you need to succeed is a really good reason to change and that takes two things: knowledge and motivation. Knowledge is what you are getting when you read this book. You also get health knowledge from public service announcements on TV, wellness programs, health newsletters, health articles, media outlets, videos and health documentaries. You are reading what I, the expert, have to say about good health. As far as you know I could be making all of this up. But I have no reason to lie to you, plus I'm really just the messenger. The end of this book has a list of references I've used to document where all this information comes from. If you don't believe me you can always go and look up these articles and see for yourself. Hopefully I have earned some of your trust, but trust is hard to come by these days. Most of the information you and I hear or read is tainted by those with a financial interest in the information. Today, it is harder than ever to find accurate health-related information that is free from marketing deceptions, conflicts of interest and outright lies. I have another friend who is taking a supplement to lower his blood cholesterol. He has learned from his neighbor that a certain supplement is all natural, 100% pure and effective at lowering blood cholesterol. What his neighbor didn't say is that he's part of a multi-level (or pyramid) marketing company that promotes a great way to earn money from home while selling supplements. His neighbor makes money every time a person buys the supplements. Without good research, it is impossible to know if the supplement has any effect on cholesterol or any dangerous side effects. The reason this gentleman is taking this supplement is because his neighbor convinced him it would be effective at treating his high blood cholesterol. Hopefully, no harm will come from this, but more than likely no good will come either. If you have fair, unbiased information you can use that knowledge to come up with a really good reason to change. Of course, where can you get unbiased health information?

A few years ago I reviewed over 1,000 research articles as I wrote the national bestseller, *The Culprit & The Cure*. This book shows the why, what and how of healthy living. It is based on research from the world's best and brightest health researchers. It is still a very accurate and unbiased source of health information that provides readers with the knowledge to successfully change behaviors. Others also take this unbiased approach to providing health knowledge to the public. Most sources of health information that come from the federal government are generally free from many of the biases that can alter the truth. Health information from federal agencies, major universities, community organizations and not-for-profits is generally very accurate when you contrast this information with those who have a financial interest in the topic. If non-profits and government groups are on one end of the accurate information spectrum than pharmaceutical companies, food manufacturers and restaurants are on the other end of the spectrum.

Take the Chobani yogurt company for example. They produce fruit-flavored Greek style yogurts. Don't get me wrong, I like yogurt but what really bothers me is how they manipulate the truth. Next time you are at the store pick up a container of Chobani yogurt and look at the ingredients. The number two most common ingredient is evaporated cane juice. What in the world is evaporated cane juice? It's just a fancy way to say sugar. Chobani is extremely good at marketing and selling yogurt. They know health conscious consumers will avoid foods that contain the word sugar. So, they just replace the word sugar with evaporated cane juice, which sounds a lot healthier. Chobani is in the business to make money and they are going to manipulate the truth in any way they can to get you, the consumer, to purchase more. Your knowledge about the health benefits of consuming yogurt is tainted by those who want to sell a lot of yogurt.

Chobani is not the only food manufacturer who's going to bend the truth to gain financial favor. We've already covered this topic in earlier chapters, but in order for you to have a really good reason to change you need to have truthful information. Food producers are perhaps some of the worst sources of untainted health information. Nutraceutical and supplement makers don't have to back up their health information or claims with any evidence; they can say whatever they want providing the ultimate example of "buyer beware."

A conflict arises when our desires for good health information meet the aggressive marketing and propaganda of organizations with a financial interest in making sure you get the health information they want you to have. We see this every day in politics where one side distorts the facts to their advantage while the other side does exactly the same thing. The truth is probably somewhere in the middle between the two positions. This is one reason why we are encouraged to get a second opinion regarding medical decisions or health information. The Internet makes it a lot easier for us to get different opinions. Recently, I purchased an iPad to help me stay connected while traveling. This device makes accessing the web simple and convenient no matter where I am. It's like I have the total sum of all human knowledge at my fingertips. My ability to learn and gain knowledge regarding my own health or anything for that matter has increased exponentially. With access to the web, I can gather information from multiple sources. I can compare and contrast and make a decision on whether or not what I'm learning is accurate. Now, when I think about having a good reason to change, I know that the reason for changing is based on good, trusted and accurate information. A lot has changed now that I have access to all that knowledge. My doctor hates me because I already know what I have and what the treatment should be before I ever step into her office. I just need her to sign off on the prescription. My plumber and air-conditioning professionals hate me because I stopped calling them. Any problems I have can now be easily fixed by watching a couple of videos or reading a few blogs. Accurate knowledge is power and with that power we get good reasons to change our lives. Combine your reason for change with the right kind of motivation and little by little you will start to win the battle for better health.

The Right Kind Of Motivation

Earlier I said that one of my behaviors was growing a garden. I've learned a lot over the years and my knowledge regarding the health benefits of fruits and vegetables has encouraged this behavior, but that's not the main reason why I garden. I'm motivated to grow a garden because I like the taste of the foods it produces. Back in Chapter 4 we talked about buy, taste, crave and repeat. There, we learned how our brains interpret our feelings, tastes, smells and surroundings to produce a sensation we call pleasure. When we eat a food that really tastes good our brain records this as a pleasurable experience; something that should be repeated. We also talked about how commercially available foods from stores and restaurants maximize our pleasure by carefully combining lots of salt, sugar and fat. I described this connection between our food and pleasure as buy, taste, crave and repeat. However, when we are talking about my behavior of growing a garden this saying can be modified to GROW, taste, crave, and repeat. I grow delicious tasting foods in my garden, but when the summer season ends and all of my fresh vegetables and fruit have been eaten I actually get a little bit sad knowing that it's going to be a while before I can have fresh fruits and vegetables again. My cravings persist throughout the year and I have even built a greenhouse to try to grow fresh tomatoes during the winter (notice I said try). I grow the delicious food, and when it's gone I crave it until spring rolls around and I can plant my garden anew. My behavior of growing a garden is driven by the pleasure sensors in my brain. My motivation for continuing to grow a garden every year is really just my response to some neurochemicals that have been released in my brain and make me feel pleasure. Almost every behavior that we have has a chemical connection to our brain. Some might call this neurochemistry, but I like to call it motivation.

In reality, our motivation is way more complicated than how I just described it. Sure, I like the taste of my fresh tomatoes, pears and peaches, but there's more to it than just the taste of the produce that I grow. I also have the impression that the food I grow in my garden is somehow tastier and better for me than the food I get at the store. Some of my motivation comes from the fact that I get to enjoy the wholesome act of connecting with the land in some small way. But there's more. Usually I have fresh produce for several months during the summer when my children are out of school or back from college. My family also enjoys the delicious taste of the fresh produce. They smile and their eyes light up when they consume a big bowl of fresh raspberries. I can almost always get a "thank you" and a big hug at the end of the day.

Remember, my brain is recording all of this just as it has my whole life, even when I was a child. As a small boy I used to get up every morning with my mother and go pick raspberries in a big garden that my grandfather used to grow. I grew up eating fresh produce from the garden. Once you've tasted a really good raspberry you will never forget the experience. In the summer it's also usually really nice weather where I live. We spend considerable time outside playing, working, entertaining and visiting. So, while all of this really enjoyable socializing with friends and family is going on, we are all enjoying ripe tomatoes, fresh melons and a host of other fruits and vegetables. It's kind of like a celebration of life—all of which is carefully organized and stored in my brain as a clear example of pleasure—something to be repeated again, and again, and again. So, I'm extremely motivated to grow my garden. My reasons for doing so are pretty obvious to most of you by now. This is just one example of how motivation can have a direct impact on our behaviors.

All behaviors that promote good health have a similar list of motivators. These motivators are really just benefits; the reasons why we do what we do. At the very end of the last chapter I illustrated how changing your lifestyle can really improve your health and quality of life. I talked about a large study I conducted with 365 people who demonstrated amazing improvements in their health risks after just six weeks of healthy behavior change. There's something else you need to know about the people who were in this study. They were motivated and ready to change their lives. Most of them were between the ages of 30 and 65 and most of them had gained considerable weight or had been told by their doctor that they had elevated health risks. For the first time in their lives, many of them were starting to feel the early effects of aging and chronic disease. They were aware that they had some problems. They knew that their behaviors probably weren't what they should be and they had reached a point in their lives where they were ready to act. They knew enough about the connections between poor behaviors and poor health that they wanted to do something about it. The intervention we used in this study provided them with the skills they needed, but motivation is the single most important ingredient of the behavior change secret sauce.

My motivation for growing a garden comes from my desire to repeat the pleasure I get when I consume delicious fruits and vegetables with family and friends in beautiful summer temperatures. These are what I call positive motivators—reasons for maintaining behaviors that are associated with pleasure as compared to reasons for maintaining behaviors that are associated with fear. Pleasure versus fear is what we get when we motivate people with carrots or sticks. With the carrot approach, we can motivate people by treating them with something pleasurable—a reward that means something to them. With the stick approach, motivation is achieved through fear. Both are real motivators and valid reasons to change behaviors. There's still a lot of debate about which one works better. I think there is a time and a place when fear can act as a good motivator, but those times are rare. When fear is used as a tactic to change it often works in the short-term, but it usually doesn't last very long.

A few years ago the U.S. Air Force was struggling with a high number of new recruits who were smokers. They decided to see what would happen if they forced all new recruits to stop smoking. During the six weeks of basic military training all new recruits were forbidden to smoke; any recruit caught smoking during basic training would be severely reprimanded.[3] It was believed that fear would be a sufficient deterrent to not only keep the new recruits from lighting up, but to also encourage them to permanently abstain from using tobacco after basic training. As might be expected, during the six weeks of basic training the number of recruits who smoked dropped to zero. None of them wanted to get caught for going against direct orders. For a short amount of time fear was effective at getting people to alter their tobacco use, but what happened after basic training paints a very different picture.[4, 5] Some of the new recruits who stopped smoking during basic training were able to permanently abstain from using tobacco, but most did not. As soon as basic training was over and the ban was lifted the majority of recruits who were smokers renewed their use of tobacco. The most interesting part of the study is what happened to the recruits who never used tobacco in the first place. Eight percent of the recruits who had never smoked started smoking for the first time after basic training and 43% of ex-smokers (recruits who had quit smoking before entering the Air Force) started smoking again. This study of 26,000 young men and women showed that forcing people to adopt a healthier, safer behavior can have a short term impact, but without the right kind of motivation change is fleeting.

Recently, I was contacted by a large manufacturing company in the state of Wisconsin. They called to ask me if I could help them with a problem they were having with their employees. The employer and its 800 employees shared the cost of health care. The employees paid $250 every month for health care, while the employer paid an additional $1,000 per month. The company also offered an employee wellness program, but only a few of the employees were participating. So, the company decided to link the amount employees paid for health care to participation in the wellness programs. Participating in the wellness program was not mandatory, but if you failed to participate you were responsible for the entire cost of your health care—an additional $1,000 per month. It didn't take very long for all of the 800 employees to figure out that if they wanted to save $1,000 every month they better participate in the wellness program. As you can imagine participation in the wellness programs jumped to 100% in the first month. The company was able to demonstrate great program participation, but after a year of using this approach they discovered that very few employees had healthy behaviors. Moreover, the company was seeing increases in the number of health risks and health care costs among its employees. The use of fear (having to pay an extra $1,000 every month) as a motivator worked well to get people to participate, but it had very little impact on the real problem—unhealthy behaviors.

Fear can be helpful as a motivator in some settings. Individuals who work at dangerous jobs must follow specific safety rules. If they fail to follow the safety procedures and behaviors they could be fired or worse, killed. In this case, the fear of losing a job or the fear of being permanently injured or killed can be motivation enough for some people to adopt safety behaviors at work. You and I do the same thing every day when we avoid some behavior that has previously caused us to experience fear. For example, we know that we can get hurt when we play with fire or if we touch something that we know is hot. Fear is not so much a motivator as it is a deterrent. We try hard to move away from fear and towards things that bring us pleasure. Not to sound sexist, but sometimes men can be a little bit stubborn and thickheaded. More than with females, males tend to be better motivated by fear. For example, a man who is obese may not care if his physical appearance is not what he wants, but he might be motivated to change if he knows he is likely to suffer from heart disease or early death.

A saying I heard many years ago has always stuck with me, it goes like this, "A man convinced against his will is of the same opinion still." In other words, if you use guilt or fear to get someone to change behaviors, he or she might do it but they'll do so grudgingly. They are being forced to do something they don't want to do. In this case, the motivation to change is coming from other people, not the person who's demonstrating the wrong behavior. They don't own the reason to change. The reason to change is coming from someone else and if they do make behavior change, it's not based on free will. This scenario is just like what the employees of the manufacturing plant in Wisconsin faced. They participated in their wellness program not because they wanted to but because they had to. This type of motivation does not help create a sustainable healthy culture.

Own Your Motivation

This brings us to an important point. The source of the motivation that we need to change behaviors is important. If it comes from anyone or any place outside of ourselves it may not give us reason enough to make behavior changes that can be maintained. A lot of people are fortunate enough to work at companies and work sites that offer incentives for healthy behaviors. If these employees exercise regularly or eat a healthy diet or lower their health risks they can earn financial rewards, gift cards or a discount on their health insurance costs. These types of rewards can be effective at getting people to start a healthy behavior, but usually once these incentives go away, so too do the healthy behaviors. The motivation for doing the behavior in the first place is based on some external reward like extra cash or a T-shirt or a paid day off. This reminds me of some incentives that were used by a big law firm on the east coast. The firm wanted their lawyers and all the employees to get healthy, so they started a wellness program and asked every employee to take a 20-minute health risk assessment. If they completed the assessment they got a check for $500. Not surprisingly, just about everybody finished the health risk appraisal and got their money. When the next wellness activity was announced the very first thing everybody asked was, "How much money do we get?" It turns out that the employees had no interest in really improving their health; they were just interested in how much money they would receive for participating. Since their reasons to change were based on an external motivator (money) nobody improved their health behaviors or health risks. If you and I are going to be successful at keeping our unhealthy culture from impacting our health behaviors we have to have powerful, long-lasting reasons to change—reasons that come from within.

There's nothing wrong with giving people rewards or incentives for good behavior, so long as those rewards eventually cause the person to experience the internal, personal benefits that can come from demonstrating the right behavior. When I was young I liked to run. I ran lots of road races, charity races, and even a few marathons. It was nice to get awards and a few ribbons, but what really motivated me then was the thrill of competing and pushing my body to do something I didn't think was possible. It was also kind of fun. So, my exercise habit started out with external rewards, but along the way my motivation for running changed. My reason for maintaining a lifestyle that included regular physical activity transitioned from external rewards toward more internal motivators. I now exercise every day because I like the way it makes me feel. I feel better when I exercise, I sleep more soundly and I use exercise to break up my workday so that my mind has some time to rest and think about other things. I exercise every day because I think it makes me more productive. As I age, my regular exercise keeps me from feeling stiff and sore. My lifetime habit of getting regular exercise has nothing to do with my fear of getting chronic diseases or premature death, even though these are very real benefits that I stand to gain. I don't exercise to keep my blood cholesterol low or to decrease diabetes risk. I have a good diet and I don't have elevated health risks. Fear plays no part in my motivation for being regularly physically active; my motivation focuses on the internal, positive benefits that I receive. No one gives me a new water bottle or new running shoes or even a discount on my health care premiums. I get no external rewards whatsoever, and yet I continue to do it every day if possible because the internal benefits are all the reward I need. Exercise gives me pleasure.

Think about your reasons for wanting to change your behaviors. Where does your motivation come from? Does it come from a benefit you want for yourself—from within you or does it come from an outside source like a cash reward or pressure from someone else? Both sources of motivation are good, but motivation that comes from within us is even better. When we talk about winning the battle for better health and counteracting the unhealthy culture that surrounds us you should consider all of the benefits that await you. I like to focus on the positive ones like spending more time with my grandkids, having good health later in life that will allow me to serve my community or church, having good enough health and quality of life to travel, see other places or just work in my garden. I'm really not afraid of death and disease as much as I'm hoping for a long, active, high-quality life with those I love and care about. This is what motivates me to push back against all the pressures that are encouraging me to live an unhealthy lifestyle. It's these enjoyable aspects of life that compel me to control how much I eat and help me arrange my schedule so that exercise is an important part of my daily life. When you combine these motivations with the pleasure I experience when I engage in healthy behaviors, the likelihood that I will maintain these behaviors well into the future is very high.

Decision Time

With good knowledge and reasons to change, the decision to engage in a healthy behavior won't happen until you decide it's worth it. There are lots of benefits I get from my garden, but growing a garden also has some downsides. It takes time, hard physical labor, regular watering and lots and lots of weeding. If it were really easy, more people would do it. To be sure, every behavior has a similar list of pros and cons. The pros are the benefits you get—your reasons for change—and the cons are the things that make it hard to change. Our unhealthy culture makes it extremely easy to adopt poor behaviors. Today, we are all in a hurry. We have little free time and disposable income. The reasons to be unhealthy are often greater than the reasons to be healthy. When we do a head-to-head comparison of the pros and cons of adopting healthy behaviors, the cons will often win out and our health loses.

Exercise Is Not Worth It

After giving a presentation on healthy living to a group of engineers in New Jersey one of the engineers shared an interesting observation with me. He was considering his motivations for wanting to get more exercise. We had talked about the results of one study that demonstrated that those who exercise regularly live about 2.5 years longer than those who do not exercise. He had calculated that if he added up all the time people spent exercising during the course of their life, they would have spent about two full years exercising. With his analysis in hand he was prepared not to exercise because he figured that the time spent exercising was equal to any increase in the length of his life. Mathematically, it was a wash. This guy was exactly the type of person I want designing bridges and cars, but not making health recommendations. He had carefully considered just one of the many benefits of exercise. His comparison wasn't a fair comparison. His list of exercise pros focused on just one benefit of regular exercise (living longer) when in reality we know that exercise offers practically countless benefits.

By now you must have a pretty good idea of what unhealthy behavior you'd like to change and you probably have a good reason to change. Now it's time to do a side-by-side comparison of the pros and cons of making this change. Here is a simple list of known benefits for eating a healthy diet and exercising. There are many more benefits besides those I've listed. Feel free to add your own and be sure to include benefits that are physical, mental, emotional and spiritual.

Check the pros you would like to enjoy in your life and add any other benefits you want that are not listed.

The Pros Of A Healthy Diet And Exercise

______ have more energy

______ I like the way it makes me look

______ maintain a healthy weight

______ reduce my stress

______ lower my health risks

______ sleep better

______ prevent chronic disease

______ keep my cholesterol low

______ improve my self-confidence

______ spend time with friends and family

______ get outside more often

______ prevent osteoporosis

______ have fun

______ feel better

______ others: ____

Now consider a few of the cons, and remember to include any others not listed.

The Cons Of A Healthy Diet And Exercise

______ it will take extra time I don't have

______ I'm not comfortable exercising

______ I really like the taste of unhealthy foods and don't want to give them up

______ I only have enough money to buy fast food

______ I don't like to sweat

______ I have small children

______ I live in an unsafe neighborhood

______ I don't have any exercise equipment

______ I don't like the taste of vegetables

______ others: ____

Neither of these lists is complete. If you carefully consider your reason to change, you can likely think of several more pros and cons. Go ahead and write them down. This will help you consider what is really at stake if you change behaviors. When you have your full list of pros and cons, consider which list is the most important to you. Are the pros more important or are the cons? This process of considering the pros and cons is a great way to make sure you are really motivated to change. When you reach a point where the pros are more important than the cons, you're ready for Step 2: Learn New Skills. Hopefully you won't wait until you're 80 years old before the pros outweigh the cons.

Island Native

My name is Lesley Wharton, and I live and work in Newark, New Jersey. I'm a shift supervisor at a natural gas power plant and I am the poster child for all the middle-age women who struggle to be healthy. As a single mother, I have to balance my family obligations with my work. Thank God my mother is available to help with my kids. I sit behind a desk all day and sip coffee or diet Coke to keep me going. Over the years, I've gained some weight and picked up a few bad habits like eating a lot of fast food and not getting enough sleep. The other day, my 12-year-old daughter asked me why I was breathing so hard bringing in groceries from the car. I noticed it too. Decades of neglecting my health have taken a toll on how I look and how I feel. Her comment and my longing to look and feel healthy again were enough to make me want to change my life. I want to be able to do simple chores and not feel winded. I want to sleep better and I want to be around to see my children go to college and begin their own families. My mom has decided to join me in making some changes. I've been stuck with the same unhealthy habits for a long time, but now, I'm motivated and determined enough to do something about it.

CHAPTER 10

Step 2—Learn New Skills

SHORTLY AFTER WORLD WAR II, JAPANESE MANUFACTURERS FIGURED OUT HOW TO GRADUALLY IMPROVE THE QUALITY OF THEIR PRODUCTS. With time, Japan became known for creating high quality products and equipment. A key component to their success was making small, meaningful improvements over time. This same process is also a very effective way to think about human behavior change. Healthy behaviors that are maintained for a lifetime almost always start with baby steps. When compared to someone who's trying to change several behaviors at once, those who take baby steps are much more successful. Research studies have shown that people who make small, manageable changes in their lives are more likely to maintain those new behaviors as compared to those who try to change everything at once.[1]

Most people these days can be pretty impatient; they want good health and they want it now, not six weeks from now or six months from now. Because of our impatience, many of us try to do too much too quickly, which can lead to failure. There's something special that happens when we take small steps in an effort to have life-long health improvements. In this chapter, you will pick which behavior you want to change as well as the tools or skills you will need for success. But you only get to start on one at a time, even if you have numerous habits that you would like to change. Like the Japanese manufacturers the best outcomes happen when people make small, continuous improvements. When you take a small step to improve your health, such as eating more fruits and vegetables every day, the odds of successful behavior change go way up because every successful small step actually changes your brain.

Let's say you decide to eat more fruits and vegetables every day. After a week of trying you realize that you actually did it—you were successful at making a short-term change to your diet. This is a success. Granted, it's a small success, but a victory nonetheless. As you think about the change that you have just made your brain will store the emotions, thoughts and feelings you had in the pleasure centers of your brain. That little step of changing your diet for just a few days has created a positive memory and experience that is now stored in your brain. Contrast this with an unsuccessful attempt to change several things all at once. For example, suppose you wanted to eat more fruits and vegetables every day for a week, exercise for 35 minutes every day for a week and stop eating sugar. Because you have daily demands on your time and energy, your initial determination to change will help you succeed for a few days, but eventually you may find it harder and harder to stick with it. Chances are by the end of the week you will have failed to change all three behaviors. And just like in the first example, your brain is recording all of your emotions, thoughts and feelings. Only this time it doesn't get stored in the pleasure centers. Everything gets stored in the, "I can't do this. I'm not strong enough" part of your brain. Ouch, nobody needs those memories. In fact, these negative memories and emotions can sabotage your efforts to get healthy. That's why I like the idea of taking baby steps. With small changes we experience small successes, and we feel positive emotions that our brains label as pleasure—something to be sought after and repeated.[2] When we have mastered one small behavior change it's time to take on another until we have mastered several healthy behaviors. By taking small, manageable steps we create positive experiences over time. Eventually, our health improves and we will have created our own culture of health.

At the end of each chapter in this book I have shared personal stories of people from all over who have taken the "baby step" approach to healthy living. I call them Island Natives because they all have created and live in small islands of health. It is fun to read their stories, but the Island Natives provide us with more than just some interesting personal stories. They show us how to navigate the journey to better health. I call this learning wisdom from the wise. They can tell us what to avoid and what to do to be successful. However, they are not the only ones who have been able to create and live in a new culture of health. There are large groups of people who have been successful at losing weight and keeping weight off for decades.[3] There are also groups of people who were sedentary and have been successful at becoming fit.[4] We would be wise to learn from those who have successfully blazed the trail to better health. It would be even better if we could learn the same skills and tools that they use to be successful.

Skills And Tools

We've talked about our reasons for change and about our motivations for change, but most people want to know, "How do I do this?" The how of behavior change includes learning new skills and having the right tools. Everyone is certainly different, they don't all use the same skills and tools, but they do use something. It takes some skill to be healthy. Learning to shop for healthy foods is a skill. Knowing how to cook a healthy meal is a skill. Learning to hit a golf ball straight down the fairway is a skill. Skills are abilities to complete a task, and without the right skills we may not have the ability to carry out a healthy lifestyle. But don't worry, none of this is complicated—anyone can learn the skills required to have a healthy lifestyle.

Along with some new skills, it's helpful to have the right tools; things that make being healthy easier to do. It's easier to walk on a regular basis if you have a pair of comfortable shoes. The shoes in this case are nothing more than a tool, something that makes it easier to be healthy. Here are some common tools people use to be healthier: a healthy recipe book, a cutting board to cut vegetables, a fast food nutrition guide, a membership to a local gym, a planner to schedule exercise, a stroller for your baby, a bicycle, a set of golf clubs, home exercise equipment, a shopping list, a pedometer to measure your daily steps, a shovel to help you grow produce in your garden…you get the idea. Tools are the various things we need to help us be healthy. Different health behaviors have a different set of tools. For example, the tools you need to get better sleep, such as a dark room, and a comfortable bed are not the same tools you would need to decrease your alcohol consumption. And just like trying to do too much at once can lead to failure, trying to use too many tools at the same time can make changing behaviors way more complicated than it needs to be.

I'm not the only one who recognizes the importance of having the right tools and skills to help change behaviors. In his book, *In Defense of Food*, Michael Pollan provides a very simple list of strategies that anyone can use at any time to make healthier food selections. Here's what Michael suggests:

1. Look at the ingredients in the foods you eat. Avoid foods that contain ingredients that are unfamiliar, unpronounceable, more than five syllables long or that include high-fructose corn syrup.
2. Shop the outside aisles of the grocery store (that's where the produce and whole foods are)
3. Shop at a farmer's market or produce store
4. Eat more like the French, Italians, Japanese, Thai, or Greeks
5. Don't get your fuel from the same place your car does.

I especially like the last one, "Don't get your fuel from the same place your car does." The next time you go into a convenience store try to find a food that your great grandmother would recognize. No doubt about it, gas stations and convenience stores are ground zero for all foods full of salt, sugar and fat. None of these foods were available 50 years ago. Most are highly processed, full of unpronounceable ingredients and packed with calories. If you talk to any of the Island Natives discussed in this book, you quickly learn that they have learned not to buy any foods at the same place that they buy gas. This one skill alone will help you improve your health.

The five strategies that Michael suggests are more important than you might think. If we talk to those who were wise, those who have already been successful at adopting and maintaining healthy behaviors, almost all of them probably follow these strategies. They are simple, easy to remember and they work. Additionally, there are many other different tools we can use to eat healthier, be active, lose weight and create a healthy culture.

Inside The Aldana Home

I consider myself and my family to be Island Natives. Even though we live in the United States and see the same food marketing that everybody else does we have been able to create a healthy culture in our home. Once in a while we eat out, but it is a real challenge to eat foods outside the home that are still healthy. We've become very selective about the restaurants we visit. In some ways, eating at a restaurant is more like trying to find the best of the worst from a selection of really unhealthy foods. Once in a while I might have an Egg McMuffin and a glass of orange juice from McDonald's. Sandwich places such as Blimpie's or Subway can provide a pretty healthy sandwich. Occasionally, we will eat at Panda Express, an Asian fast food restaurant located in some parts of the U.S. The food there isn't perfect, but it is one place where I can get a big serving of fresh cooked vegetables that really taste good. Our favorite restaurants are some of the international foods such as Thai, French, Japanese and Mediterranean. Generally, they are made with fresh vegetables and contain very little salt, sugar and fat. We like the taste of Thai food so much that we've learned to make many of the recipes at home. More importantly, all of my children and grandchildren have learned to enjoy a variety of Thai dishes. They like the taste and the food is good for them. We've been successful at making delicious Thai recipes because we have some tools that help us. It is important to have the right ingredients, so we often visit a local international grocery store. I also have a wonderful Thai cookbook that was given to us as a gift. Its pages have been soiled, folded, torn and thoroughly enjoyed. With the right tools we've created a healthy food environment that is enjoyed by all of our family.

Skills And Tools You Need To Eat Healthy At Home

If you don't exercise at all you can likely live for decades, but if you don't eat at all you'll soon be dead. Everybody has to eat to survive. The real challenge is deciding what to eat and where to get your food. Think about where you get your food. If you eat at home, the food you are putting in your mouth has come from a garden, grocery store or restaurant. If you are traveling, you will likely consume food sold in airports. Some people get the food from their workplace vending machine or cafeteria. If you are still school-aged you probably eat food from your school cafeteria. Depending upon the source of the food there are different tools and skills you can use to make healthier food selections.

My company, WellSteps, offers several different behavior change campaigns. One of our campaigns is called "Food Makeover." In this program, we demonstrate the different tools and skills people need to eat healthy foods at home. We start by looking in the refrigerator and cupboards for foods that are healthy and for foods that are not so healthy. To make this determination, we help you learn how to read the ingredients on labels, shop for healthy foods and how to prepare healthy meals. We call this program Food Makeover because we show people how to remake their food environment.

Healthy recipes are another tool that can help you maintain a healthy diet. There are many recipe books to choose from. So long as they use whole foods and stay away from a lot of salt, sugar and fat you're probably okay. I have spent years collecting healthy recipes that I like. All of them can be found at **wellsteps.com/recipes** and they are free! I encourage you to look through these recipes and try cooking something you've never tried before. You might be surprised by the delicious taste and I guarantee you'll be eating healthy.

I also like to let my children participate in preparing meals. Once a week or so each child gets to choose what we make for dinner, but they can only pick healthy meals. They also have to help cook. We spend quality time together, and they get great pleasure out of determining what healthy meal we eat.

Besides healthy recipes, we have other tools that we use in our home. We have a rice cooker. It's awesome. You take some brown rice, rinse it off, add water, push the button and you are done. In a few minutes the rice cooker cooks the rice and automatically shuts off and keeps it warm for you. You can purchase an automatic rice cooker for about $15. Other tools that make eating healthy include a blender (for fruit smoothies), cutting boards for chopping lots of vegetables and a barbeque for grilling fish and lean cuts of meat. Many people use automatic bread makers to make fresh, whole-grain bread. One year I got really crazy and bought a small apple press. Every fall we harvest our apples, grind them up and press them until delicious apple cider comes out. We store the cider in half gallon plastic bottles and freeze them. All winter long we enjoy delicious apple cider. I agree that not everybody is going to press their own apples, but we do. It's good family fun and we enjoy the delicious juice.

Not long ago I decided to make some Thai lettuce wraps. The recipe calls for ground pork, lots of spices and vegetables. I had no idea what I was doing so I used one of the best tools I have for healthy eating: the Internet. With very little effort I found a free video that showed me exactly how to make Thai lettuce wraps. I watched the video and within just a few minutes I created a healthy meal that impressed my children so much that I got several "thank you's" and hugs. Videos, recipes and how-to articles available on the web today make it easier than ever to eat healthy at home.

Where You Get Your Food

The food you cook at home has to come from somewhere. Most of it probably comes from a grocery store, but people are increasingly getting their food from farmer's markets, community gardens and their own gardens. If you don't grow a garden you can buy produce from those who do. At **localharvest.org** you can type in your zip code and find all the farmer's markets and local produce stores in your area. Never before has it been easier to get fresh produce at reasonable prices. When you buy produce that is grown locally you support your local economy, you help protect the environment and you get to eat fruits and vegetables that are at their peak of freshness and taste. There's nothing quite like a fresh garden tomato to put a smile on your face.

Skills And Tools You Need To Eat Healthy At Thc Grocery Store

The biggest source of food in the American diet is the local grocery store. Selling groceries is big business; it's also an old business. For decades, the grocery industry has been carefully studying how consumers make purchasing decisions. This has become a hard-core science with treatment groups, control groups and sophisticated statistical analyses. You may not know it, but when you walk into the grocery store you are seeing decades and decades of research on how to get you to purchase as much food as possible. Everything from how and where food is displayed to the actual layout of the store has been carefully designed and created to maximize the amount of food you will purchase. When you walk into a grocery store you are at the mercy of the owners of that store and food producers they represent. Earlier in this book we discussed the deceptive practices and outright lies food producers use to convince you to purchase their products. Indeed, the grocery store is where much of our unhealthy culture is allowed to flourish. Fortunately, with the right tools and skills it is possible to make the grocery store an ally rather than an enemy of good health.

Try this little experiment. Next time you are in a grocery store, take a look at what's in other people's grocery carts. Don't think of it as spying; think of it as doing field research. I do it all the time, mostly out of curiosity. If you find a cart that is filled with fresh produce, whole-grain breads and other healthy foods chances are very good that whoever is pushing that cart has a very healthy lifestyle and you will be able to see the effects of that healthy lifestyle on how they look. They probably look healthy. On the flip side, if you find a shopping cart that is filled with highly processed foods that contain a lot of salt, sugar and fat chances are that the person pushing the cart will look differently. There's a lot of truth to the saying, "You are what you eat." This saying is never more obvious than in the grocery store. Remember, some people are also looking in your grocery cart, wondering about the different kinds of foods you eat. Those who know me know I'm a healthy guy. My life today is surrounded by the food police—people who know me and know what I do for a living. They are always carefully inspecting the foods I purchase to make sure I don't buy anything deemed to be unhealthy. As long as I'm working to improve public health, I'm destined to be scrutinized by the food police. Luckily, I don't mind, most people are just having fun.

Stop & Go At The Grocery

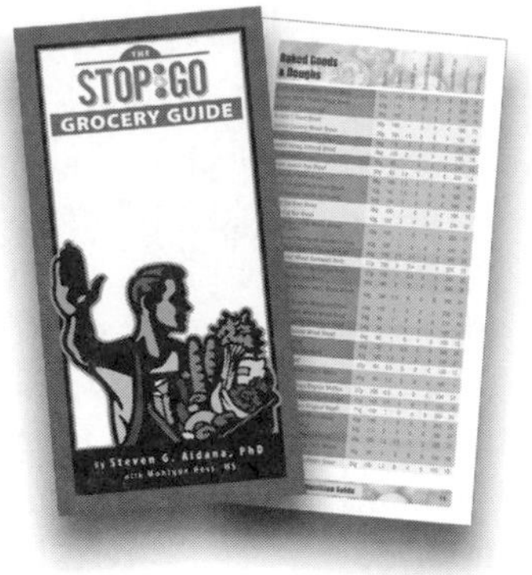

Take a look at the ingredients listed on the foods you're considering purchasing. If the food contains ingredients that are unfamiliar or unpronounceable or that contain high-fructose corn syrup try to find a healthier option. This is not easy to do for most people. That's why we created *The Stop & Go Grocery Guide*. Several years ago we acquired several grocery food databases. There are over 300,000 different foods that can be purchased in grocery stores. No wonder it's so hard to find the healthy foods! We gathered nutrition information on the top-selling 3,500 foods in the United States. Then we used a team of nutrition experts and a simple set of rules to classify every one of these foods according to their nutritional value. There's nothing magical about these rules except they give some indication as to whether or not a food is close to or far from its original form. From these rules, a red, yellow and green color-coding process was developed. *The Stop & Go Grocery Guide* is a tool to help people successfully navigate the grocery store maze. With this guide you can easily see which foods are the healthiest. There is a printed version of the guide and even downloadable apps for both iPhone and Android devices. You can learn more about these at **www.fastfoodbook.com**. This grocery guide is one tool to help you make healthy grocery purchases.

A Few Words On Costs

Does healthy food cost more than unhealthy food? This is a question I hear all the time. The answer is yes. Food close to its natural form like fruits, vegetables and whole grains cost more than foods that have been highly processed and have added salt, sugar and fat. The high cost of healthy food is just one of many barriers that keep us from purchasing healthier foods. In reality, the calories our bodies get from food has never been cheaper. Mass production of highly refined carbohydrates and flours that contain added sugars and fats make the average cost per calorie very low. College students, struggling single-parent families and those who have fallen on hard economic times likely eat a diet that is different from those who have more disposable incomes. Ramen noodles, boiled potatoes, bread and cold cereals purchased in bulk are all examples of relatively inexpensive foods that provide a lot of calories for a very low price. On a cost-per-calorie basis food is a bargain.

When you purchase a soda that has free refills, you can get a lot of calories for very little price. These foods provide a lot of calories but little else because they are low in nutrients, phytochemicals and have few health-promoting values. One dollar can buy 1,200 calories of potato chips, but just 250 calories of vegetables and 170 calories of fresh fruit.[5]

Foods that are close to their natural form like fruits, vegetables and whole grains are full of nutrients. They are also more expensive. A study in the state of Washington showed that the poor spend about $6.77 per day for food while those who are better off economically spent almost twice that much. A comparison of the nutrients between the two groups showed that the poor consume more calories, more fat and more sugar, but far fewer nutrients like potassium and iron. In the United States poor families spend less money on food, but they eat more calories while those who have more money are able to purchase healthier foods, which have fewer calories and more nutrients.[6] In the U.S. we have built a food system that favors calories over nutrients, and thus there is an enormous supply of cheap calories.[7] This system is a big part of our unhealthy culture. This system is directly responsible for the fact that the highest rates of obesity can be found among people with the lowest incomes and the least amount of education.

There is additional proof the U.S. food system is to blame. In third world countries poverty is almost always associated with failure to thrive nutritionally, muscle wasting and emaciated bodies, but here in the U.S., poverty is associated with excessive weight and obesity rates that are the highest in the nation. The difference between the two is a food system that favors calories over nutritional content. The less money you have for food the more salt, sugar and fat you consume, which complicates the desire to eat healthy. If you are poor and the only foods you can afford are low-nutrient foods full of salt, sugar and fat, the addictive properties of these ingredients will influence your taste preferences, and reinforce your desire to purchase low-nutrient, high-calorie foods. This problem can be summarized like this: Lack of education and lack of income cause us to purchase high-calorie, low-nutrient foods that taste delicious and cause obesity. The states with the highest rates of obesity are also the states with the lowest income and education levels. This is not a coincidence.

So what do we do about it? What tools can we use to fight against this cultural trend that has such a tight grip on so many of us? There are really two problems here. The first is the fact that healthy food costs more and the second is that inexpensive, unhealthy food has a greater appeal to our sense of taste.

Tools & Tricks Of The Trade

There are several tools and skills people have used to overcome the high cost of unhealthy food. These tips come from people who have been successful at adopting and maintaining healthy behaviors.

Be Careful With Coupons

Even though you may be tempted to get a good deal, be very careful with coupons. Most coupons offer discounts to highly processed foods with questionable nutrient value. Don't be tricked into purchasing foods with the coupon if those foods are not at or near their original form. To help cut costs, plan your meals ahead of time by preparing healthy recipes that can be used for more than one meal. Healthy leftovers are an inexpensive option for good nutrition and a sound budget.

Watch For Sales On Healthy Food

Watch for sales of healthy food and when they happen, buy in bulk. There are some healthy cold cereals like Wheaties, Wheat Chex and other whole grain cereals that don't contain sugar. They can be expensive if you don't get them on sale. When they do go on sale, buy enough to last the entire year.

Buy Foods That Are In Season

Fruits and vegetables are cheaper when they're in season. They are also cheaper when purchased at a farmer's market.

Consider Canned Foods

Fish is healthy, but pretty pricey when you buy fresh. You can buy fish that's been canned and still get the same nutrition for a lot less. Anytime you buy fruits and vegetables that have been frozen, canned or even dried, they usually cost less. This is especially true when they are on sale.

Grow Your Own

Finally, one of the least expensive ways to get whole foods is to grow your own.

But what about overcoming the delicious taste of those cheap, inexpensive foods? I think this is an even more important question than just the cost alone. Foods close to their natural form should be part of our new lifestyle, but obviously they taste different than highly processed foods loaded with salt, sugar and fat. If you don't really like the taste of vegetables it's time to start experimenting with new ways to cook vegetables. I've already mentioned my ability to cook delicious Thai dishes. I had to learn how to cook these recipes, but along the way I overcame my dislike for vegetables when I discovered how delicious they could be. Experiment with some new recipes. Purchase fruits and vegetables when they are in season and you might be surprised at how delicious they really are. Most of the fruits and vegetables at the store were picked way before they were ripe—it's no wonder so many people don't like the taste.

Something else happens when you start down this journey to better health. When you start to replace unhealthy foods with healthier foods, your taste preferences will change. There are foods or candies that you used to eat when you were a child that you no longer like. For me it's suckers. When I was a kid I liked suckers—I liked the taste. Now that I'm older I no longer have the desire to eat them; whatever appeal they had to me when I was younger has completely disappeared as my taste preferences changed. This is similar to the enhanced taste sensations that ex-smokers talk about after they quit smoking. While they were tobacco users they had dulled their sense of taste. However, without the tobacco their taste buds are able to finally sense each and every flavor food has to offer. When we consume healthier foods we get introduced to a whole new world of taste sensations and soon our preferences will change so much that we no longer will like many of the foods that we consumed in the past.

Skills And Tools You Need To Eat Healthy At Restaurants

In 2007, I convened a panel of nutrition experts to review the nutrition content (salt, sugar and fat) of every single fast food offered by the nation's 70 most popular fast food restaurants. The panel was asked to review all 3,500 foods and code them red, yellow and green based on their nutrition quality. The colors of the traffic light are easily understood by all, and since we were not conflicted by pressures to serve the food industry we were brutally honest with our recommendations. Red foods should be avoided, yellow foods require caution and green foods are the best. I like to think of the green foods as being the best of the worst because most fast foods are not foods in their natural form. They are foods that have been highly processed and infused with salt, sugar and fat. Even the green foods are not ideal, but they are considerably better than the foods coded red. The final product was a guide called *The Stop & Go Fast Food Nutrition Guide*. I made a printable PDF copy of the book available for free at **fastfoodbook.com**. Almost 100,000 people downloaded the PDF, and people kept asking for a professional printed copy so we put it in a book format. We even made an app for both Apple and Android devices. Since then, over 500,000 copies of the book have been sold.

Once all the fast foods were color coded we could identify the restaurants with the best and worst foods. Think about all the different types of fast food restaurants that surround us. They sell pizza, tacos, hamburgers, fried foods and many other foods. Of all the different fast food places can you guess which ones provide the most foods that earned the red badge of shame? The worst of the worst are the breakfast food restaurants like Denny's, IHOP and Waffle House. Based on the amount of saturated fats, sodium, processed meats, and lack of whole grains and fruits and vegetables, the breakfast restaurants are the worst places to eat. Based on our nutrition rankings, here is a rough guide to the best and worst fast food restaurants:

WORST

Breakfast specialty	Denny's, Waffle House, IHOP
Traditional fast food	Burger King, KFC, McDonald's, Chick-fil-A
Mexican	Taco Bell, Del Taco, Taco John's
Italian	Sbarro
Pizza	Pizza Hut
Healthy Asian foods	Panda Express
Sandwich shops	Subway, Blimpie's, Boston Market, Panera

BEST

Think about fast food restaurants that serve meals that contain fruits and vegetables. Sometimes it's is hard to think of any, but the sandwich shops and a few others do. They get recognized for having the highest number of green colored foods. Any restaurant can offer a few healthy options: McDonald's serves apples and IHOP serves green beans, but the rating system we used took an average of all the foods they offered.

I don't have any scientific proof for this next point, but it seems to me that people who eat a lot red colored fast foods or who eat a lot of meals at some of the worst restaurants are also many of the same people who are struggling with body weight and diabetes. And the opposite is also true—people who eat a lot of green colored fast foods or who eat a lot of meals at some of the best restaurants are NOT struggling with excessive weight and diabetes. You can test this idea yourself. Go have a meal at Denny's, IHOP or Waffle House (well maybe not a meal, maybe just a cup of coffee). While you are there, look around at who else is eating there. You might see one more glaring example of "you are what you eat."

It is almost impossible to live in our American culture and not eat fast food. We have found that there are people who do occasionally eat fast food and also maintain good health. They may use one of the *Stop and Go Nutrition Guides* or they may use other tools to stay healthy. When we ask healthy people what tools they use to eat out and still stay healthy we discover that they share some common tools:

- When you want popcorn at the movies, order the smallest size and don't get free refills.
- When eating out, share a meal with someone. These days, serving sizes are so big they can easily feed two.
- Don't hesitate to leave food on your plate and take the rest home for leftovers. (I like the shredded pork salad sold by a small restaurant chain called Café Rio. The meal is so large I get full after eating less than half and I take the extra home with me. Most often I can get three meals out of one order).
- Avoid extra calories by drinking water every time you eat out.
- Select vegetables any time you are given a choice.

One of the worst food environments we face is our modern airports. Travelers often arrive hungry and pressed for time. If you travel often you know it is especially difficult to find healthy foods while traveling. Early in my career, I started to have opportunities for business lunches and dinners that were held at nice restaurants. Some years, I would take well over 100 business trips a year. On any of those trips, I could order anything I wanted from the menus. It didn't take long for me to figure out that if I wasn't careful I could easily become the unhealthy culture poster child. It was during these years that I became a master at using the healthy eating tools and strategies we've been discussing.

A few years ago I received a letter from an inmate at a federal prison. He had read my book *The Culprit & The Cure* and wanted to tell me about the tools he had used to eat healthy while in prison. Unlike you and I, prisoners have very little control over their food culture. Most prison food could be considered adequate for survival, but not typically conducive to long-term health. This inmate told me that while in the cafeteria, he noticed some inmates were getting meals that contained large servings of fish, fruit, vegetables and whole grains. He was told these were special meals for Jews and Muslims. Knowing he had a sentence of many years and wanting to get access to healthy foods, he concocted a plan to convince the guards that he was Jewish. He memorized the Jewish holidays, met with the prison Rabbi and professed his conversion to Judaism. On one hand I was disappointed to learn of his fake Jewish conversion. I don't think it is appropriate to lie about such things, but on the other hand I appreciated his ability to manipulate the prison system to get healthier meals. Soon, he was eating three very healthy meals a day. He went to great lengths to create a healthy culture, even as an inmate in federal prison. The point is this: If this guy can create a healthy culture in prison, you and I should be able to do it as free citizens.

Skills And Tools You Need To Exercise

People who get regular exercise and enjoy all the benefits of being active are use different strategies and tools to help them stay active. Typically, when we think about exercise tools we think about exercise equipment such as treadmills, weights, golf clubs, bicycles, snowboards, tennis rackets, and a variety of exercise clothes and accessories. All of these are nothing more than tools that help us remain active. In addition to these tools, you undoubtedly need some skills. To be sure, without the right skills and tools it's unlikely to get the benefits of regular physical activity. I often get asked what I think is the best type of exercise for people to do. People who ask this question are hoping I'll say something like cross-country skiing, yoga or running. I tell them that the best type of exercise is the type you like to do the most. Whatever form of exercise you like to do on a regular basis is the best type of exercise for you. For some people it's running and for others it's walking. Despite how many calories are burned per minute or what muscle groups are strengthened, the only thing that really matters regarding your health is finding physical activity that you like to do. All the exercise equipment and tools in the world are of no value if they don't get used. You can buy a gym pass, get special exercise training and buy nice workout clothes, but if you don't use them you won't experience the health benefits of exercise.

Of all the different tools and strategies that can be used to help us get regular physical activity there is one that is especially important: time management. In our fast-paced society there are a lot of demands on our time. Work, sleep, travel and relationships can take up the entire day leaving little time for regular physical activity. These are the top priorities of our lives that have to be attended to. However, the need for regular exercise will never go away, so the challenge is to find time for exercise that can fit in and around our priorities. When we talk about time management I often think about the past few presidents of the United States. These are perhaps some of the busiest people in the world and there are huge demands on their time. And yet, despite their tremendous work responsibilities all of our recent presidents have made regular exercise a priority. They have made time to be physically active despite their incredibly busy schedules. If they can make time for exercise there are very few excuses for you and I.

If you are still struggling to find the time, there are several strategies you can use to make time to be active:

- Include exercise with other activities that you have to do. For example, have a business meeting while going for a walk or exercise with family members.
- Don't think of household chores or yard work as burdens, rather think of them as opportunities to be active.
- Rather than use the elevator or the escalator, take the stairs.
- Walk or ride a bike to a nearby appointment or meeting.
- If you're traveling, walk to your terminal as opposed to taking a shuttle or moving walkway.

Each of these strategies works because they involve including regular physical activity into a normal daily schedule. Unfortunately, my job requires that I sit at a desk all day. Because I'm sedentary at work I have to find opportunities at work to be active. Although being active during the day while at work helps with my fitness, it's not enough exercise to get all the health benefits. In addition to finding opportunities to exercise during my work day, I also have time during the week dedicated for exercise. Before or after work, on most days of the week, I will either go for a walk or ride my bicycle and I'm almost always with a family member or my dog. Two or three times a week, I also do some strength training exercises for at least 30 minutes. I have realized that the time I spend getting regular exercise provides not only benefits to my health, but it makes me more productive when I am at work. It sounds counterintuitive to spend time exercising when I could be working, but the time spent moving my body is time well spent. The benefits I get are truly astounding. If the presidents of the United States find it important to allocate time during their schedules to be active they must be receiving benefits too.

I've been able to make exercise a priority in my life, but I also have some tools that help me. I have a decent pair of walking shoes, and I have a bicycle, helmet, and riding clothes that I wear when I ride. I even have an old iPod so I can listen to music during my long rides. I also have some 30-pound dumbbells that I like to use when I lift weights. I bought them at Walmart—they didn't cost much and they work great. I've been able to make time to be active, but I also have a few tools to help me enjoy it. I can still exercise without the tools, but they do make it easier for me. Some people like to use exercise videos, fitness classes, walking clubs, exercise equipment, pedometers, and/or iPods or iPhones with various exercise apps and calorie counters. I see a lot of people walking while they're doing business on their cell phones. All of these tools can be helpful if they are used. Unfortunately, just about every home in America has some form of exercise equipment that was purchased with good intentions but no longer gets used. If you're thinking about buying a piece of exercise equipment look for equipment that's used, that way you can give it a try without spending as much money.

Weight Loss Tools

The tools we talked about for eating healthier and getting exercise are the same tools used to control body weight. For years, I have been saying that weight loss and maintaining a healthy weight are really just a side effect of a healthy diet and regular exercise. After all, our body weight is largely determined by the number of calories we eat and the number of calories we burn. A weight scale is a great tool to help you monitor your weight. I recommend people weigh themselves often. The information we get from the scale doesn't lie. It provides an unbiased, unemotional appraisal of your weight. If you choose not to use a scale to measure your weight about the only other way you can monitor your weight is to see how your clothes fit or to look at yourself in the mirror.

There are some very good calorie counting programs on the web and on mobile apps. I don't have the patience to count all the calories that I eat. And since I eat a healthy diet I don't worry about calories. That being said, I do know people who use these tools to effectively keep track of how many calories they have consumed throughout the day. Using a free web-based calorie counter or app can certainly help you reduce the number of calories you consume every day and subsequently lose weight. If you think this might be of value to you, give it a try.

It's time for you to start eating better and exercising more. Below, I've listed all of the tools and strategies that were discussed in this chapter. Based on your motivations and reasons for change, you now get to select the tools and strategies you think you can realistically use. Look at each of the tools and mark the ones that appeal to you. Remember, don't try to do too much at once. Pick just a few that you are confident you can use. You can even set a goal for yourself. As you start to make progress toward your goal, enjoy your small victories and remember them. This will help you stay motivated.

Some of you may be looking at this small number of weight loss tools I've listed and wonder if there are more tools you can use to control your weight. Your body weight is directly impacted by all the diet and exercise tools we've already talked about. In reality, they are also weight loss tools. Pick some and use them and you'll start to impact your body weight.

Pick the tools and strategies you can use to eat healthy:

- Look at the ingredients in the foods you eat. Avoid foods that contain ingredients that are unfamiliar, unpronounceable, more than five syllables long or that include high-fructose corn syrup
- Shop the outside aisles of the grocery store (that's where the produce and whole foods are)
- Shop at a farmer's market or produce store
- Eat more like the French, Italians, Japanese, Indians, Thai or Greeks
- Don't get your fuel from the same place your car does
- Go to **wellsteps.com/recipes** and try some new, healthy recipes
- Have your children help prepare healthy meals
- Buy a rice cooker, cutting board or blender to make healthy foods
- Use the Internet to find healthy eating videos and recipes

- Visit **localharvest.org** to see where you can buy locally-grown food
- Get a free copy of *The Stop & Go Fast Food Guide* at **fastfoodbook.com**
- Be careful with coupons; use them only for healthy foods
- Make large servings of healthy meals and save the leftovers for later
- Buy healthy foods in bulk when they're on sale
- Get fruits and veggies cheaper when they are in season
- Grow your own fruits and veggies
- Get and use a copy of *The Stop & Go Grocery Guide* at **fastfoodbook.com**
- If you get popcorn at the movies, order the smallest amount and don't get refills
- Share a meal when eating out
- When eating out, leave food on your plate and take the extras home
- Drink water instead of juice or soda
- Select veggies when given the choice

Pick the tools and strategies you can use to exercise regularly:
- Select a strategy to manage your time
- Include exercise with your other "must do" activities
- Treat chores and yard work as opportunities for exercise
- Take the stairs
- Walk or ride a bike to meetings or appointments
- Make time during the week for exercise
- Buy exercise tools, equipment or electronic devices you know you will use
- Get and use a weight scale
- Try using a calorie-counting website or app

Island Native

My name is Lucinda, and I'm a lawyer in Phoenix, Arizona. Like a lot of people, I got a good job and spent the next 20 years sitting at a desk. Responsibilities that come with my job have to be balanced with my family responsibilities. I had children of my own and had to help care for my aging parents. Both my father and mother have become type II diabetic and the last time I had a checkup I discovered that my blood sugar was a little bit high. Not wanting to become like my parents, I decided it was time to do something about my health. I started by talking with my doctor and my husband about what I needed to do. Even though I have never struggled to maintain a healthy weight I still had an elevated risk for developing diabetes. The number of calories I was consuming every day was not a problem; it was the quality of my food and my lack of exercise. So, I started making small changes in the foods I was eating. Rather than eat highly processed foods like white bread, baked goods and desserts I started eating foods closer to their natural form like vegetables at dinner and a piece of fruit for breakfast. More importantly, I changed my daily schedule so that I could walk every day for 40 minutes before leaving for work. Every morning I get up, put on my walking clothes and walk for almost three miles before I have breakfast. I'm much more selective about the foods that I eat and every time I eat out I make sure I'm having some type of vegetable. Although I haven't lost any weight (I didn't have any to lose) the last time I had a checkup, I found out that my blood glucose was in the normal range. All I needed to do to stop the development of diabetes was become more active and make small changes in my diet. I'm now 46 years old and I've never felt better.

CHAPTER 11

Step 3—Help From Others

LET'S TALK ABOUT THE LAST AND PERHAPS MOST IMPORTANT STEP NEEDED TO HAVE A HEALTHY LIFESTYLE AND CREATE A HEALTHY CULTURE: HELP FROM OTHERS. I'm going to give you a few illustrations to help you see why help from others is so important to our success. Picture a typical, middle-aged male. Let's call him Larry. Besides the cost, taste and convenience of food, what else determines what Larry eats every day? Most likely, Larry shares his life with others such as a spouse, family members and friends. If Larry is like most middle-aged males, he may not spend much time shopping for food and preparing meals. This work is likely being performed by a spouse or partner. If Larry is going to be successful at eating a healthy diet, he is going to need help from the other important people in his life. Without support from friends and family it is very unlikely that Larry will be successful at adopting and maintaining a healthy diet. In this example, help from others refers to receiving support and motivation from those with whom we live.

Another way of thinking about help from others is to consider how our immediate environment can help or hinder our efforts. When my children were younger we lived in the Midwest. We had a modest home, a big yard and a safe neighborhood in which to play. We had created an environment for our family where healthy food was always served, sedentary activities were limited and the children were encouraged to spend a lot of time outside playing. We had created an environment that supported a healthy lifestyle for all of us. Some friends of ours had planned a vacation and needed someone to watch their 10-year-old son while they were gone. Since we had children who were about the same age and plenty of room we agreed to watch him for two weeks. This boy came from a home environment where physical activity was not encouraged and food was not as healthy as it should be. He was also 20 pounds overweight. For the next two weeks, this boy was exposed to a very different environment. When his parents returned after their two-week vacation they were shocked when they saw their son. By eating healthier foods and having an active, fun lifestyle he had lost quite a bit of weight. Our healthy home environment had a great impact on him during the two weeks he spent with us. Interestingly, within a couple of months the 15 or so pounds that he lost while at our house had all come back. In this example, help from others refers to getting help from our immediate environment. It's easier to be healthy when our environment encourages us to make healthy choices.

The last aspect of help from others has to do with rules or policies that make it easier to be healthy. Earlier in Chapter 8, I mentioned that 12% of the adults in the state of California smoke, while smoking prevalence for the rest of the United States is around 23%. This begs the question: Why are there so fewer smokers in the state California? The difference is almost entirely due to the smoking rules and policies found in that state. It is illegal to smoke in public places like parks or beaches in California. Voters in the state of California have passed laws that limit where tobacco products can be used. They have made it hard to use tobacco. And because it's hard to use tobacco, many people have decided to quit.

State and local governments, employers, and municipalities can create policies and procedures that support healthy behaviors. These policies are very effective at helping people change behaviors and maintain healthy lifestyles. Of course, you and I don't write and implement policies. We don't even use the word "policy" we usually use "rules." We make rules at home, with our children and for ourselves to help us make better decisions.

To be successful at having a healthy lifestyle we need help from others in the form of close friends and family, changes to our environment and creating and following rules that promote good health. By the end of this chapter you will have learned specific strategies on how to get support from others, how to change your environment to make being healthy easier and how to implement rules that support your efforts.

Environment Is Everything

You are ultimately responsible for the food you put in your mouth and for getting regular physical activity. Even though you have this ultimate responsibility, when you live in a culture that is so dominated by unhealthy food options, unsafe neighborhoods and limited opportunities for physical activity your freedom to make responsible choices is greatly diminished. Even if you want to make healthy choices it may not be easy to do. Your ability to have a healthy lifestyle is limited when you're surrounded by rules and environments that make it hard to do so.[1] I like to look at it like this: my diet, exercise and smoking behaviors are greatly influenced by my family and friends, my immediate environment and the policies, rules, and laws that influence me. All three elements have a direct influence over my health behaviors and that influence can be good or bad.[1]

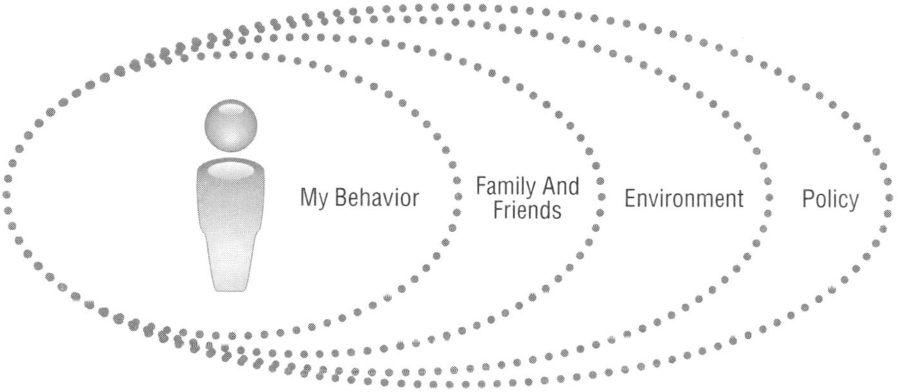

Every choice that we make and every behavior that we choose is influenced by our surroundings. Some of the biggest influences come from our family and friends.

Support From Others

My grandmother lived a very healthy life and had keen sense of humor. As we celebrated her 104th birthday, she commented that she had outlived all of her neighbors and friends and that for the first time in her life handling pressure from peers was easy because all her peers were dead! I laughed, but realized that others with whom we share our lives have a large effect on us. Spouses have a particularly large influence. Individuals who are married or enjoy close relationships have a direct influence on each other. Couples tend to share resources, materials, income and behaviors. With time, couples begin to live and act like each other. You can measure the health risks and health behaviors of one person in a relationship and accurately predict the health risks and health behaviors of the other person in the relationship.[2] That's because couples have a tremendous influence on each other.

Say you are in a relationship and you decide you want to change your lifestyle and maybe lose some weight. When you lose weight, your partner will generally do the same, without even trying. Your dietary and exercise changes will affect your partner's diet and exercise habits. You will likely both lose weight because you greatly influence your partner.[3] This is true when you're trying to adopt healthy behaviors, and sadly it's also true if one partner adopts negative behaviors. If one partner starts eating an unhealthy diet, smoking or being sedentary the other partner is likely to do the same. One study assessed the health behaviors of newlyweds just before marriage and for several years following marriage. The longer the partners were together the more similar their health behaviors, health risks and lifestyles became.[4]

So how exactly does a spouse or partner influence your behavior? My wife and I have a division of labor in our home. I do a lot of the cleaning and she does most of the shopping and cooking. Because she does much of our food purchasing and preparing she also controls what the rest of us do or don't eat. A lot of homes have an arrangement where one person is primarily responsible for making sure people are fed. Researchers call this person the nutritional gatekeeper. Studies have demonstrated that the gatekeepers influence 72% of the food their family eats.[5] If my wife, the food gatekeeper in our home, wants fewer sweets and desserts, we all get fewer sweets and desserts. If she wants to cook more fruits and vegetables, we all get more fruits and vegetables. If she wants to go for a walk, the dog and I are generally obliged to go with her.

Her decisions affect my health and my decisions affect her health. Behavior change specialists know the importance of having help from spouses and significant others. When we started WellSteps, our employee wellness company, we decided very early on that if we were going to be successful in helping employees change behaviors we would need to engage their spouses and significant others. When a company uses our programs to help their employees improve health the employees' spouses and partners can also participate. The encouragement, motivation and interest that comes from spouses and significant others is one reason these programs improve health.

Social support is the most powerful among strong and close relationships. As opposed to peer pressure, which can come from anyone at any time, you are much more likely to be influenced by your spouse or best friend. You are also influenced (albeit not as strongly) by more casual relationships such as social groups, teams, church groups and even pets. All of your relationships can provide social support to help you be healthy.

Several of the behavior change programs we do at WellSteps are team-based. Individuals get support and approval from team members who are all engaged in the same activity and working towards the same goals. Communication between family members, groups or teams can provide substantial motivation to keep you on task and to make you work a little harder. Indeed, we are more successful at changing behaviors when we work together as groups. Groups like Alcoholics Anonymous (AA) and Weight Watchers have been using social support and group dynamics to motivate and encourage people who are trying to change behaviors. Each and every one of us has an influence (good or bad) on those with whom we share our lives. Though you may not know it, you are influencing and being influenced by the people you associate with. This was very clearly demonstrated by researchers who evaluated how obesity is influenced by our social networks.[6] If a person in this study had a friend who became obese that person's chances of also becoming obese increased by 57%. If an older sibling became obese, the chances of the other sibling becoming obese increased by 40%. If a spouse became obese, the likelihood that the other spouse would become obese increased by 37%. Keep in mind that these effects were not seen among neighbors in close geographic locations, but rather only among people who had social relationships. These results were independent of the fact that some people who became obese might select close friends who were also obese. There's no doubt about it; we become like the people we associate with because we learn to share the same cultural and lifestyle habits.

Let me share a quick story to illustrate this point. One of my employees graduated with a Master's degree in health. She had a very healthy lifestyle. Not long after starting to work for us she married a nice young man who did not share her same healthy lifestyle. His entire family had unhealthy lifestyle habits; almost all of them were obese and almost all of them were developing type II diabetes. Every time she would join her husband in family gatherings she was amazed at how everybody in the family shared the same unhealthy food and exercise behaviors. Little by little, she began to introduce her husband to a different, healthier way of living. It took several years before he exchanged his unhealthy diet with a delicious, healthier one. Now both of them enjoy the benefits of good nutrition and a new culture of health. Her relationship with him gradually altered his lifestyle. Unfortunately, his family has not changed their unhealthy ways and to this day they all continue to gain weight and develop chronic diseases. Happily, she was able to help him make small changes to his lifestyle, but it could have gone the other way. Had she not been committed to her way of living she easily could have been assimilated into his family's unhealthy culture where she too would have started down the path to obesity and chronic disease.

How To Get Support From Others

Here is a simple list that can help you tap into the critical support you need in your life. To maximize your success in changing behaviors use just one or two of these ideas:

- Ask a friend or family member to join you in your journey to better health. Tell them what you are planning to do and how you will be changing your life and invite them to change with you.
- Get an exercise partner or buddy; even your dog can make a great exercise partner. After you find an exercise buddy exercise together as much as possible.
- Eat healthy meals with friends and family. Ask family members or friends to help cook and prepare the meals. Kids who eat healthy meals at home will grow up to eat healthy meals later in life.
- Enter a competition or share a fitness goal with a friend or family member. You'll keep each other accountable and the friendly competition can fuel motivation.

Environment

As you read this book, take a minute to look around you. What you see is your environment. Your health behaviors are influenced by what's in your immediate surroundings. If you are at home, your environment includes everything in your house, including your kitchen and yard. Your home environment also includes the neighborhood and community in which you live. If you are at school or work, your environment includes everything that surrounds you, including the neighborhood. Our immediate surroundings influence our behaviors.

To drive this point home, I want you to pretend you work at a desk all day. What would happen if someone placed a bowl of chocolate on your desk? If you had an enormous amount of self-control you might be able to abstain from the chocolate, but if you're like most people you're eventually going to have some. Now, how much chocolate would you eat if there was no chocolate near you? Probably none. In carefully controlled studies, people ate an average of 2.2 more candies each day when the candies were nearby.[7] The further the candy is from the person the less of it they eat. Having candy within our reach undoubtedly prompts us to eat more. Even if you can't see the candy, but know it's there you will eat more of it.

Unhealthy food in your environment—whether you can see it or not—increases the likelihood that you will eventually eat it. Fortunately, the exact same thing is true for healthy foods. If you have fruits and vegetables in plain sight more of them will be eaten.

Every day we live, work and eat in environments that influence our behaviors for good and bad. In a very real way we are a product of our environment. Those who are successful at creating cultures of health have shown us that it's much easier to be healthy when we live, work and play in environments that support a healthy way of living.

I have the privilege of working with the California Health and Longevity Institute (CHLI) in Thousand Oaks, California. The Institute provides healthy living programs for individuals and businesses. Every year I help train business professionals on the importance of employee wellness programs. I get to stay at the Four Seasons hotel which is part of the Institute and eat the delicious food provided by the staff at CHLI. The food is always extremely delicious and very healthy. Every time I'm there I eat like a king and am confident that I'm having a very healthy meal. It's practically impossible not to eat healthy while I'm there because the environment they have created surrounds the guests with so many healthy food options. The Institute understands the importance of healthy living and gives everyone who enters their environment a chance to actually practice healthy behaviors. I really enjoy my work with the Institute, but my environment there is not like the environment everywhere else. Only the rich and famous have private chefs who can prepare delicious meals that not only taste good but are also very healthy.

Sleeping and eating at the California Health and Longevity Institute kind of reminds me of the people who participate in the popular television program *The Biggest Loser.* In this program, individuals who are morbidly obese work in teams to see who can lose the most weight. They have full-time chefs who prepare healthy meals for them and they spend hours in the gym working with personal trainers who help them get fit. The people on the program live at "The Biggest Loser Ranch" where they enjoy an environment that makes it easy to be active and provides foods that are not only healthy, but that also taste good. Just like CHLI, The Biggest Loser Ranch is a great place to practice being healthy. Of course, for those of us who live and work in the real world it is unrealistic to expect that this kind of healthy environment will automatically be created for us. If we want this type of healthy environment, we will have to do it ourselves.

No one is going to show up and magically remodel our environments so that they are more conducive to better health. All of us have to work hard to create the environments that will support our healthy behaviors. These include the environments in and around our homes, schools and places of work. Here are some strategies that many of our WellSteps clients have successfully used to create and sustain environments that help them stay healthy.

Build A Moat Around Your Home

You are more likely to eat unhealthy foods if you know they are in the house. In most cases it's best not to bring these foods home in the first place. Foods high in salt, sugar and fat are usually the ones that tempt us and cause us to gain weight. My wife considers these foods to be "contraband" foods that contribute to poor health and/or weight gain. Metaphorically speaking, we have built a moat around our house. It's a simple strategy for better health that says if a food is not good for us we shouldn't buy it and bring it home. If it's not in the house, it doesn't get eaten. It's really pretty simple. If you don't buy it you won't eat it. It is a lot easier to be healthy when you look around the kitchen or refrigerator and only see foods that contribute to good health.

Assess Your Home Environment

Take a minute to complete this simple assessment of your home environment. Below are the environmental strategies that contribute to a healthy environment and lifestyle. Check the strategies that apply to you, and give yourself a pat on the back—these are excellent strategies and if you're completing any of them you're on the right track!

Good Environment Strategies

- I eat at least one vegetable with my dinner on most nights.
- I usually eat a piece of fruit with my breakfast.
- My fridge has vegetables that are cut-up and ready to eat.
- The only bread in my kitchen is whole-wheat or whole-grain.
- Most of the cereal in my pantry is whole-grain.
- The only type of pasta I buy is whole-wheat pasta.
- If I cook rice, I use brown rice or a brown/white blend.
- When I cook vegetables, I either stir-fry them with healthy oil or I steam them.
- I only bake with whole-wheat flour or a whole wheat/white flour blend.
- I set out my exercise clothes before going to bed so it's easier to exercise the next morning.
- I know if and how many fitness centers are near my home.
- I know what walking and jogging trails are in my community.
- I experiment with exercising at different times of the day.
- When possible, I walk instead of drive the car.
- When I exercise outside, I have the proper gear for the current weather conditions.

Now do the same thing for the not-so-good strategies listed below—check the items that apply to you.

Not-So-Good Environment Strategies

- My fridge has high fat dairy products such as sour cream, butter, cheese and whole milk.
- My freezer contains meats like steak, roast, pork, sausage, bacon or hot dogs.
- My pantry has many different types of chips, cookies and crackers available for anytime snacking.
- One shelf of my fridge is dedicated to soda pop.
- I usually keep at least two cartons of ice cream on hand.
- I have cured meats in my fridge such as bologna, hot dogs, bacon, sausage and pepperoni.
- When I eat toast, I always use butter or margarine.
- I only exercise outside when the weather is perfect.
- I exercise at night, outside, by myself.
- When I run or walk, I have to run in the street.
- I always use the elevator to get to my home or office.
- I don't exercise because none of my friends or family likes to exercise.

After completing these assessments you should have a good idea of what you're doing right and where you need some improvement when it comes to your home environment.

In addition to our homes, many of us spend a good amount of time at a worksite each day. In fact, many of us spend more time at work than any other single location. Since our work environment has such a strong influence on our behaviors there are strategies we need to use at work to make it easier to be healthy. We don't have the same amount of control over our worksite as we do at our homes, but we still have some. At WellSteps we created a tool to help you assess your work environment and the tool also offers ideas on how to go about creating a healthy work environment. This tool is called the Checklist to Change and you can access it by clicking "Tools" on **WellSteps.com**. Along with this tool, you can work with your boss or human resources department to create a healthy environment at work. While working with your managers and worksite leadership you'll likely find that there are other employees who would appreciate some healthy options at work. Use the Checklist to Change to identify strategies and policies that are good and not so good at your work environment. As you begin to create a healthy worksite environment you'll find it gets easier and easier to be healthy, and before you know it you will have created a healthy environment and a culture that supports good health and a high-quality life.

Your Community Can Help You

Every neighborhood and community has local government officials. Most communities also have a parks and recreation department. Do a web search or contact your local government to learn about parks and trails in your area. Communities that have invested in trails, bike lanes and walking paths are among the healthiest communities in the country. Don't just take my word for it; watch people who are using your parks and trails. You'll see people who are taking advantage of a supportive environment and who have healthy lifestyles. Use the trails as often as you can—you'll get some great exercise and you'll be rejuvenated just by being outside. If you don't have good trails in your neighborhood or community, contact your local government and volunteer to help the area organize and build trails.

The city of Fort Collins, Colorado has one of the most extensive trail systems in the country, providing over 280 miles of bike trails. You can go just about anywhere in the city using these safe, automobile-free trails. Even if you don't have a bicycle you can check one out from the city library for free. The city of Fort Collins has created an environment that supports healthy behaviors and they have a healthy population to show for it.

Rules Can Help Us Be Healthy

Every day 32 million children in the United States get free or reduced price meals while at school. For decades the food industry has exerted tremendous influence on the foods that are served to our children, and they eventually turned healthy school meals into a diet full of salt, sugar and fat. Now one in three children in America is overweight or obese and half of our children will be type II diabetic by the age of 40. To prevent the early deaths and suffering that will come to those who gain weight at such an early age, First Lady Michelle Obama worked with congress to pass the National School Lunch Program under the Healthy, Hunger-Kids Act of 2010. For the first time in decades this new law requires schools to serve more fruits, vegetables and whole grains. These rules are completely voluntary for schools. The schools are free to serve anything to their students, but if a school wants reimbursement from the federal government for those meals it must follow the new rules.

This is the first time in decades that any changes have been made to the school lunch program. Some food manufacturers are very unhappy with the changes and have asked their congressman to stop the act. Others feel that the new requirements will help reduce obesity among our children, save lives and prevent unnecessary suffering from chronic diseases. This is an example where the federal government has adjusted an existing policy in an effort to improve the health of Americans.

Recently, the New York City Board of Health voted eight to 0 to make it illegal to sell sugary drinks in cups larger than 16 ounces.[8] Any restaurant or movie theater in New York that dispenses sugary drinks cannot sell more than 16 ounces of it at a time. Sugary drinks, like soda, have been shown to be a major contributor to excess body weight and obesity in the United States. Although this is an effort to improve public health, many view the actions by New York City as an example of city government gone bad—a law that introduces excessive regulation that hurts businesses.

I get e-mails and phone calls on a regular basis asking my opinion of local, state and federal policies aimed at restricting our food choices. Most of them come from people and industries who don't like to see government intruding into people's private lives. They usually ask for my opinion, but this is the wrong question to ask. In my mind the question should be, "What can and should we do to prevent the premature death and excessive suffering of hundreds of thousands of children and adults who have unhealthy lifestyles?" When the question is phrased this way, we get a different perspective on the problem officials are trying to solve. I understand this is a very emotional topic for many people. Anytime government gets involved in our lives people can become upset. I realize that sometimes well intended laws and regulations can have unintended consequences. The alternative is to have no regulation and no laws. The trick is to try to find a healthy balance between the two because no matter how much or how little regulating the government enforces, someone or some business is not going to be happy.

I think the recent changes made to the school lunch program are some of the best public health policies we've seen in decades. No school is being forced to follow the regulations because they're voluntary. Schools can decide if they want to comply, and most will because they want the money. As a result of complying, the health of millions of young Americans will surely improve. I'm not sure what effect limiting sugary drinks to 16 ounces or less will have on the obesity prevalence in New York City, but I do like the idea of trying it for a while to see what happens. If it works, and obesity prevalence is reduced, it's a great idea to be tried in other cities and if it doesn't work the NYC Board of Health should go back to the drawing board and try experimenting with other policies that might have a positive effect. This Board of Health understands the magnitude of the problem in New York City. The NYC Board is comprised of physicians and health experts who see the suffering that obesity causes. They are passionate and sincerely interested in saving lives and helping people have a high-quality life. People may not like the policies that they recommend, but you cannot fault their sincere efforts to improve public health.

Governments establish regulations and policies in an effort to improve our health and safety. Most often these policies are well intended. At worst they are ineffective and overbearing. At best they can prevent chronic disease, premature death and unnecessary suffering for millions and millions of people. Governments have successfully enacted laws and policies to fight the use of tobacco. At one point in U.S. history 51% of all Americans used tobacco, and today that number has been cut in half. Of all the tools, strategies and motivations we have to change behaviors one of the most effective strategies is the use of health-promoting policies and rules.

Inside The Aldana Home

When one of my sons was a teenager he and his friends would log into the Internet, put together a team and fight other teams in a virtual online game called League of Legends. This game is very well-designed, it's exciting to play, you can play with your friends and if you're not careful you might become addicted to it. His mother and I watched as his playing time increased from one or two hours a day to too many hours a day. This went on for some time until one night I awoke worried about the impact this game was having on his physical, social and spiritual development. The next day we had a family meeting where we introduced a new policy (a rule actually). We call it the screen time rule which limits the amount of time our children can spend playing computer games to one hour per day. This is a drastic departure from the 7.5 hours spent online by most teenagers. I knew this was not going to go over well, so I prepared a list of 101 things he could do besides play Internet games. To help enforce the rule we even temporarily changed passwords to web-connected devices he might use. Surprisingly, he understood our concerns. Implementing the screen time rule has been one of the best things our family has ever done. Rather than come home from school and spend the rest of the day online with his virtual friends we started to do things together as a family. He started playing more sports, he read some good books, he helped provide some community service for some neighbors and he started spending more time on his school work and art projects. He even learned how to cook. Simple rules in our homes can help us create a culture of health.

I have not completely given up hope that our state and federal governments might be able to help slow down and reverse the obesity trend and help all Americans adopt and maintain healthy behaviors. Changes to the school lunch program are a great step in the right direction and I hope to see more of the same. But as I have carefully studied how our unhealthy culture was created in the first place and how our efforts to be healthy are so easily thwarted by those who gain financially from our current poor health status, I am more convinced than ever that individuals, families, employers and communities are the best places to solve this problem. For every health-promoting policy and regulation being considered by governments few ever make it into law. But for every health-promoting rule and guideline proposed within families and worksites almost all of them get adopted.

Here are some rules that can be used at home to help you be healthy. Like the other suggestions made in this chapter, pick one or two that you think you can implement.

- Eat fruits and vegetables at every meal
- Don't eat after 7:00 pm
- Don't buy sugary cereals
- Have a piece of fruit with breakfast every day
- Don't buy white bread
- Exercise every day
- Don't buy soda
- Don't buy doughnuts or other pastries
- Avoid foods full of salt, sugar and fat
- Use *The Stop & Go Fast Food Guide* to make healthy selections
- Limit screen time

In this chapter I've listed a lot of strategies that can help you be healthier. I do worry that you might become overwhelmed at how complicated it is to successfully change behaviors. I'm not going to deny the fact that it is hard to change—all you have to do is look at the worsening trends in obesity to see that most people fail to make long-term behavior changes. It's not easy, but it is possible. Bookmark this chapter and come back to it again and again. Each time you look at it pick a different strategy or rule that you have yet to try. Eventually, these small efforts start to add up because you will be creating an alternate, healthy culture for yourself and your family. The more time you spend in this culture the better your health will become. You will soon discover that the little island of health you have created at your home will connect with other islands of health. As these islands start to connect we start to produce a network of interconnected people who all share a common lifestyle and desire for optimal health. It is the creation and expansion of this network that will ultimately help us all win the battle for better health.

Island Native

My name is Marisha. I'm 32 years old and I am a hospital nurse in Oakland, California. People think that healthcare professionals like me and others who work in hospitals have really healthy lifestyles. However, our work is stressful, we are always very busy and with the little free time we have to eat we don't eat very well. I'm obese and out of shape just like several other nurses that I work with. Sometimes I look around at my colleagues and wonder how we all got so heavy. I didn't look like this in college.

The management team at my hospital has also noticed our poor lifestyles and elevated health risks and decided to implement an employee wellness program. Every time we do different wellness activities we get points that save us money on our healthcare premiums. In addition to the wellness programs, a lot has changed at my hospital. They built locker rooms with showers so that hospital employees can exercise before or after work. They changed our health insurance benefits so that any preventative cancer screenings are free. They made the entire hospital campus a smoke-free zone—it's against the rules to smoke anywhere on hospital property, even in the parking lot. More importantly, they changed the foods that are served in the cafeteria. They used to have a grill and a fryer that was used to serve fried foods every day. Then, they changed it so fried foods were available only on Monday Wednesday and Friday. After six months of that, they removed the fryer altogether. Anticipating an uproar from employees who wanted fried foods the chef introduced a new selection of really healthy international meals. Every day we get delicious, healthy foods from a different part of the world. Our cafeteria is now the most popular place to eat. It has become a lot easier to stay healthy now that my worksite has changed. The employees are happier and we're all starting to lose weight!

CHAPTER 12

Win The Battle

I HAVE A LOT OF FRIENDS WHO ARE VEGETARIANS. MOST OF THEM ARE CONVINCED THAT THE VEGETARIAN DIET IS THE ONLY WAY TO HAVE REALLY GOOD HEALTH. I certainly agree that a vegetarian diet is very healthy and there is a lot of good research to support this way of eating. About two percent of the U.S. population is vegetarian. I am not a vegetarian, but I would consider myself to be almost vegetarian. I still eat meat once in a while but in very small quantities. Socially, I consider my healthy diet and the diet of my vegetarian friends to be about the same. We get strange looks from people who observe what we eat. We stand out from the crowd because we don't eat many of the foods that are culturally accepted by most people. If you eat foods that are relatively low in salt, sugar and fat you are not eating at most of the restaurant chains located in United States. That means you are forced to eat at restaurants that do not serve these foods and when you shop at the grocery store your cart is filled with healthy food selections. If you are successful at creating and living on an island of health you will probably have to get used to others watching your eating and exercise behaviors.

Some of you might know what I'm talking about. There are certain places in the United States where if you mention that you have a healthy diet and eat only healthy foods, you are going to get strange looks. I experience this all the time when I travel. When I'm working in the "meat and potatoes" places of America (states and cities where obesity prevalence is very high) I always get a strange look when I ask for whole grain bread, a salad or an extra serving of vegetables. Sometimes, it feels like I'm all alone when I order or purchase healthier foods. Usually, I'm by myself or with a group of business people I just met. This is when my individual island of health starts to get noticed by others. Often others look at me as if they were the food police, carefully observing who is eating what. They worry that I may be offended if they eat something that both of us know is not very healthy or they wonder if I approve of what they are eating. When you live on an island of health people are going to notice what you do because you're not like everybody else—you are different. Many people will support your efforts, but some will mock them. Most of the time this mocking is just an outward expression of frustration by those who want to have a healthy lifestyle, but haven't yet been able to achieve it. Those who mock you do so because it's easier to make fun of someone who has a healthy lifestyle than it is to join them. Whenever I have people expressing interest or disdain for what I'm eating I always offer to share some with them. Generally, this piques their curiosity even more.

At the end of each chapter in this book I have shared stories of individuals who have been successful at creating and living on islands of health. These island natives have been able to change their immediate environments to create surroundings that support their efforts to be healthy. I call these people Island Natives because they live on islands of health but they don't live by themselves. Every day they interact with others while still holding true to the healthy culture they have created.

As we adopt and maintain a healthy lifestyle we will begin to impact those around us like our friends and family. Even if you live alone, you are influencing those around you. Every time you purchase a healthy product or food at a store you have influenced not only the store that sold you the product, but also the food manufacturer or farmer who supplied it. Your purchase has an influence on the supply and demand of healthy foods. Every time you buy food at a restaurant you are influencing the foods that are sold at that restaurant. The opposite is also true. If you purchase foods that don't contribute to good health you are encouraging manufacturers to produce more unhealthy food. When a food stops selling stores and restaurants will stop offering them. The law of supply and demand is always trying to provide consumers with the foods they want, when they want them. When a food is not in demand, it simply disappears from the shelves. This is just one example of how your new lifestyle can influence others, and in this case, businesses.

You also have a direct influence on your friends and family. This diagram shows how one island of health—you and your desire for healthy behaviors—has a direct impact on those with whom you interact.

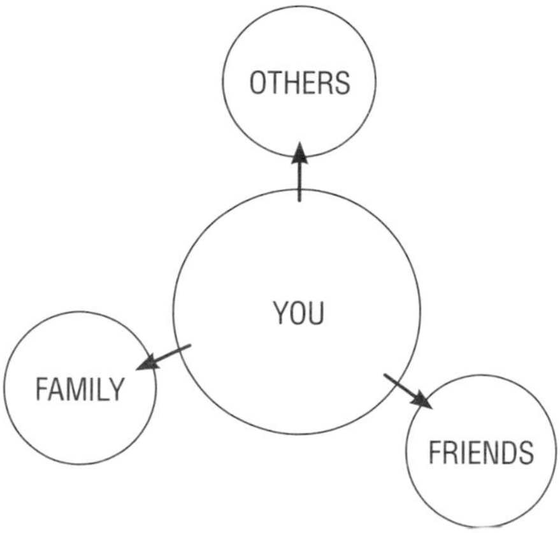

Your food choices have a direct impact on those who make a living selling food. Your lifestyle choices also have a direct impact on your family members and friends. This is exactly the way the individual islands of health start to connect. One individual influences someone else to adopt healthy behaviors who in turn influences others to do the same until a network of people with healthy lifestyles begins to take form.

These connections are happening all the time and can form in many different ways. For example, you may start to change your lifestyle by exercising and eating better. After adopting these behaviors for some time, you then attend a family gathering where people notice that you've lost weight and look healthier. This is confirmed when they see you eating small portions of healthy food. You and your healthy behaviors have just influenced close family members. They see how these new behaviors have improved your life by helping you lose weight and enhancing your health. Although most of them will go about living their normal lives, a few may want to join you on your journey to better health. At this moment, the island of health you have created for yourself is now becoming linked to another person or family member wanting to do the same. The network of people with healthy lifestyles just increased by one.

This may seem trivial, but this is precisely the process used to revitalize and transform entire communities. It is the process by which change among a few individuals can be repeated and amplified in a way that affects whole groups of people. It is the process by which culture change occurs. Once people understand how much better their lives can be when they have a healthy lifestyle more and more people start wanting the same benefits.

Any time family members get together cultural influences can be felt. This is true for the foods that we eat and it's also true for our exercise patterns. Prepare a healthy meal and share it with any friends or family and you will have given everyone a slight push towards a healthy culture. Go for a walk or exercise with someone and the two of you will be sharing a healthy culture. Go out to eat and make a healthy choice on where and what to eat and you will have influenced those who are with you to do the same. Each time you and others make a healthy purchase you provide financial support and encouragement for restaurants to offer more healthy options. When you buy healthy foods you stimulate business growth and sustainability and you are helping to alter the culture.

I have met individuals from churches, synagogues and religious communities who have created committees and church health ministries to provide healthy meals and activities for their members. One church member has organized a women's group to meet at a local church for Zumba dance and exercise classes every morning. Using church facilities this one person has now created dozens of new islands of health among the members of her church. Make no mistake about it, when you participate in a walking group, walking or running event or join a sports team you are influencing others to have a healthy lifestyle. When you work in a community garden growing fresh produce or teach others how to grow fresh produce you are expanding the healthy lifestyle network. As the network of individuals with healthy lifestyles continues to grow, people start feeling better and enjoying a higher quality of life.

The diagram below shows how you influence friends, family and others to have a healthy lifestyle. This is how it works with just one person (you). But in reality you aren't the only person trying to have a healthy lifestyle. Millions of Americans are doing exactly the same thing and each of them is influencing those with whom they interact. What this diagram doesn't show is how the network of interconnecting healthy cultures is more like a giant web that stretches all over the U.S. In some places like Colorado and Washington, there are many more healthy individuals who are connecting. In these places, the web is denser because there are many more islands of health that have connected with each other. In these places, entire communities rather than just families and individuals are becoming healthier.

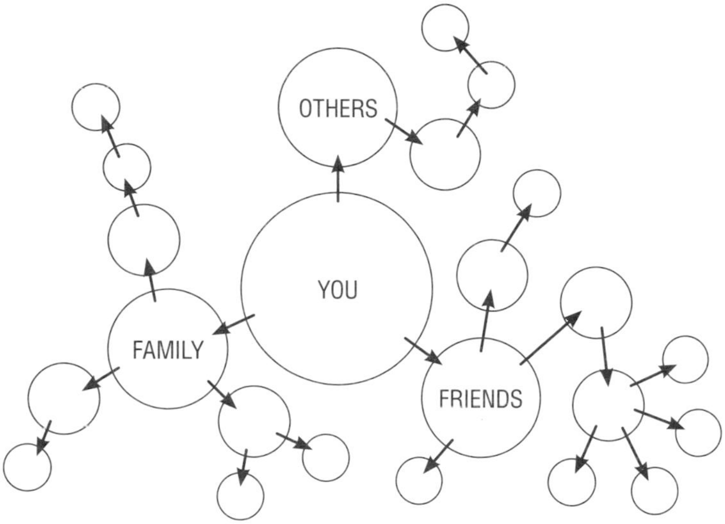

Why This Network Is Important

It is unrealistic to expect the food industry and professional organizations to suddenly offer only foods that contribute to good health. After all, they would likely lose a great deal of money with this approach. Indeed, there is simply too much money being made by those who profit from our current unhealthy culture. It is equally unrealistic to expect state and federal governments to solve this problem.

In 2010, the Executive Office of the President of the United States organized a task force to provide policy recommendations to help reverse the obesity epidemic among children.[1] This document, "Solving the Problem of Childhood Obesity Within a Generation" is packed with outstanding policy ideas that could have a very large impact on reversing obesity among children. This task force has done a fantastic job of identifying ways that the federal government can help individuals and communities create cultures of health and reduce childhood obesity. I applaud this effort, but as can be expected, powerful lobbyist groups descended upon Capitol Hill and successfully derailed the legislation proposed by the task force. When these lobbying efforts were combined with bureaucratic bickering, any hope of implementing policies to help create a healthy culture was lost. Three years have passed since these recommendations were proposed and none of them have been successfully implemented.

These well-intended, top-down approaches to improving our culture are impractical because they require political will and the ability of elected officials to resist political and financial pressure from special interest groups. It seems to me that the only viable way our culture will change is if it changes from the bottom up, starting with individuals, families, churches, employers and communities who band together to promote healthy behaviors. As more and more of these grassroots efforts come forth, our current unhealthy culture will slowly begin to change. If we're going to be successful in changing our culture it will have to change from the ground up, with individuals like you and me leading the way. It will happen person by person, family by family, worksite by worksite and community by community.

This process of improving our culture little by little has already begun. Just the fact that you are reading this book suggests that someone in your immediate circle of friends or family thinks it's important that you know this information. They know that if you implement the strategies outlined in this book you will improve your health. Whoever gave you this book or told you about it is an active participant in this bottom-up approach to our cultural transformation. And now you too have become an active participant in the transformation of our culture. Meaningful cultural change will occur when the number of people who are sincerely interested in improving their health reaches a critical mass—a tipping point where those desiring a healthy lifestyle begin to influence and connect with larger and larger groups of people wanting the same thing. When enough people express interest in changing their behaviors a movement is created. It's like a snowball rolling down a hill that gets bigger with each roll. These grassroots movements are already taking place all over the world.

As you start to improve your health and the health of your family it is natural to look at others in your neighborhood and community and want the same for them. This is exactly what Linda Fondren of Vicksburg, Mississippi did. After she created her own culture of health she began to look around at the residents of her community. Mississippi has some of the highest rates of obesity in the country and one of the unhealthiest cultures found anywhere. Empowered by her own successes and her desire to help others, she created

Shape Up Vicksburg (**www.shapeupvicksburg.com**) which is a grassroots program designed to help city residents battle obesity. She created a walking club for the entire community, started holding fitness classes and started to build bridges (in a metaphorical sense) between local health agencies, church groups and city government. Today, tens of thousands of Vicksburg residents are more active because of Linda Fondren. This is just one example of how one island of health (created by Linda) influenced others to create their own islands of health. With time, she has helped to improve the health of an entire community. She ultimately created a network of healthy communities that stretches between individuals, families, churches, community health organizations and local government. Linda is a living and breathing example of how islands of health can connect to create a new culture.

Churches can do this too. Many people are active participants in church congregations and communities. These communities can provide a tremendous amount of support for individuals and families who are working together for a common cause. As the pastor of the Saddleback Church in Lake Forest, California, Rick Warren couldn't help but notice the amount of obesity in his congregation. It became apparent to him that there was a problem when he noticed how hard it was to baptize new members of his congregation because they were so heavy. Rick was wise enough to know that if he was going to help his congregation he would need to address his own lifestyle first. Using many of the same tools and strategies found in this book, Rick created an island of health and even created a healthy living program he called, "The Daniel Program" which was based on the biblical story of Daniel and his nutritional choices. What started with one person, Pastor Rick Warren and his desire to improve his own health, expanded to include other members of his community and congregation. This is another example of how individuals can become passionate about their own health and leverage that passion to help other people. These spontaneous movements toward a healthier lifestyle are occurring all over the United States and around the world.

In major cities all across South America, community walking events are appearing. In cities like Lima, Peru you can see tens of thousands of residents out walking every Sunday. The website **www.walk21.com** has a calendar of similar walking events that are occurring all over the world. These events are not financed by special interest groups nor are they the result of local and federal government policy. They are organized by individuals who are fighting back against the unhealthy cultures that surround us, individuals who have realized that the world we now live in needs to change. These individuals are discovering that their desires for better health are not unique; many other people are ready to fight back against the culture that surrounds us.

In the French towns of Fleurbaix and Laventie parents and local officials wanted to do something about worsening childhood obesity trends among the city's children.[2] Nutritionists worked with school teachers to create cultures of health at all of the city's schools. These programs were so successful that the community as a whole wanted to be involved. They worked with restaurants to provide healthy foods, built fitness centers and established walking days. After several years, the obesity prevalence among school-aged children in these towns was half the prevalence of neighboring cities. This is an example of how culture change in schools can help create a healthier city.

Worksites Lead The Way

Nowhere are healthy cultures being created more quickly and effectively than in worksites. Companies, municipalities and corporations are very interested in improving the health of their employees because having unhealthy employees is expensive. Employees who have unhealthy behaviors generally have elevated health risks and eventually develop chronic diseases. They are absent from work more often, they get hurt more easily and they have high health care expenses. Employers are striving to create cultures of health because they need healthy employees. Sometimes they use incentives to gently encourage employees to improve their health behaviors and sometimes they are a little more forceful. I know one large insurance company that works really hard to encourage employees to be healthy. If you work for this company and you want health insurance you have to participate in their wellness programs. You can only qualify for the health insurance plan if you are willing to make an effort to have a healthy lifestyle. Participation in worksite wellness programs like this one is always voluntary, but employers want every employee to participate. Some may think that it's not fair to force employees to participate, but many companies have very few options if they want to continue offering health benefits. They need to improve employee health and spend less on health care or they won't be able to offer health care insurance at all.

Think about the last time you got insurance for your car. The insurance company asked about any previous accidents. They also obtain your car's

VIN number to see if you had any previous claims. They also use your driving history to determine how much your insurance premiums will cost. If you are a high-risk driver your insurance is going to cost more. However, if you haven't had any accidents your insurance will be less. The cost of your car insurance is based on your driving risk. Life insurance companies do exactly the same thing when calculating the cost of life insurance. If you are a smoker your life insurance is going to cost more because you have a higher risk of premature death. But it's different with your health insurance. Today, the cost of your health insurance is determined by the risk of all people under the insurance plan, not just you. For those who have jobs, the cost of health care is determined by the risk of everyone you work with. This approach is now changing, however, and many employers are now calculating the cost of your health care based on your health risk. More and more employers are beginning to treat health insurance just like auto insurance. Those with the greatest risk will pay more. To help all of us ease into this new way of calculating health insurance costs, many employers will lower your health care premiums if you participate in behavior change programs.

Back in the 70s, worksite wellness programs started as a perk for company executives. Today, almost all large corporations have employee wellness programs and they do an outstanding job of creating cultures of health. They do this by following the three steps we've outlined in the last chapters of this book. They help educate and create awareness among employees, they give them the tools, strategies and motivation they need and they provide rules and policies that help create an environment where it's easy to be healthy. The cost of having poor employee health has reached a point where most employers are willing to invest in employee wellness programs and create worksite islands of health. These programs not only improve employee health and prevent chronic diseases, but they also save money. Between individuals, families, worksites and communities, worksites have the strongest reasons to create cultures of health. Each day, more and more companies are starting wellness programs and this wave of interest may create enough momentum to help improve the health of millions of working Americans. It's accurate to say that among employers, the need to create healthy cultures at work has reached a tipping point. Successful companies that have created healthy cultures at work enjoy the benefits of having healthy employees.

A Glimpse At Your Future

Now that I have shared my vision for what it's going to take for all of us to get healthy, let me share a small glimpse into the future. As I look down the road to what the future might hold, I confess that I have no crystal ball or special ability to predict the future. What I do have is a pretty good understanding of the blatantly obvious. Let me share four future trends that are bound to continue because I see very little in the way of policy, politics or business strategy that will alter their course. I hope I'm wrong about most of these prognostications, but I'm pretty confident they are going to happen.

Trend #1: The Health Care System Will Become Unsustainable

When I was in graduate school back in the 80s there was a lot of discussion about the cost of health care. At that time, the cost of medical care had been going up dramatically each year. The average cost for medical care at that time was about $2,000 per person per year. We were all pretty convinced that the increasing cost of care was unsustainable. Today, more than 30 years later the average cost of health care per person per year in United States is around $9,000.[3] It has been increasing about 10% per year. That's almost twice as much as what in every other country in the world pays for health care. Every year, Americans pay more for health care. In 2010, Americans spent $2.6 trillion for health care.[4] Since a lot of this cost is incurred by the Medicare and Medicaid programs these two programs pose an enormous threat to the financial stability of the United States.

Here's where you come in. In the future, we are all going to pay a lot more for our already very expensive health care. It is estimated that 70% of our health care costs is due to treating chronic diseases caused by unhealthy behaviors. We've spent most of this book talking about the personal benefits that come from a healthy lifestyle. There is an additional benefit to all of us when we create islands of health. Our healthy behaviors help us have lower health risks. When we have lower health risks we have fewer chronic diseases and we use less health care. In the future, the more we create islands of health the more we will slow the increases in the cost of medical care. It will cost less because we will use less. But, brace yourself. If you think our health care system is expensive now, it's going to get worse. As the cost continues to go up there will come a time when our current U.S. health care system will become so expensive that you and I will not be able to afford it. At that point, the health care system will collapse. I'm not sure what will be created to replace it, but I am very sure that the system we have now is unsustainable. I hope I'm wrong about this one.

Trend #2: More People Will Get Healthy At Work

It's not just you and I who are paying more for health care costs. Employers are paying even more since they pay a larger share of the overall amount. For this reason alone employers have been helping their employees get healthy. In the past, employee wellness programs have only been available to large corporations. But now small and midsize businesses are rapidly implementing employee health programs. In many cases, they're doing it because they can no longer afford to provide health care benefits to their employees. Companies that have healthy employees pay less and companies that are looking to have a competitive advantage will use wellness programs as a strategy to become more profitable. If you work for an employer that has an employee wellness program they should be making it easier for you to be healthy. If the place you work does not have a wellness program contact your human resources department or talk to your boss and see if you can start one. It's a lot easier for you to be healthy if you have help at work.

Trend #3: We're Going To Get Bigger

It is my privilege to be a board member for the C. Everett Koop Health Project. Our work is to identify the best employee wellness programs in the country. Every year we review applications from organizations who are hoping to be identified as a winner of the Koop award. The award strives to acknowledge organizations who have truly created islands of health. These awards are given to only the best programs in the U.S. I am sad to admit that even among the best programs in the United States we never see behavior change programs that are able to help an entire workforce reach and maintain an ideal body weight. I've never seen a worksite or community where everybody has an ideal body weight. That tells me that even though these companies have been able to help their employees improve their health, they struggle to help all employees reach a healthy body weight. The current obesity trend within our culture is too great for even some of the best behavior change programs to overcome. On a positive note, we do see that the best programs in the country can help individuals stop gaining weight. I really believe that if we can get everyone to just stop gaining weight that would be a success.

In case you missed it, here is the obesity graph I shared with you at the beginning of the book.

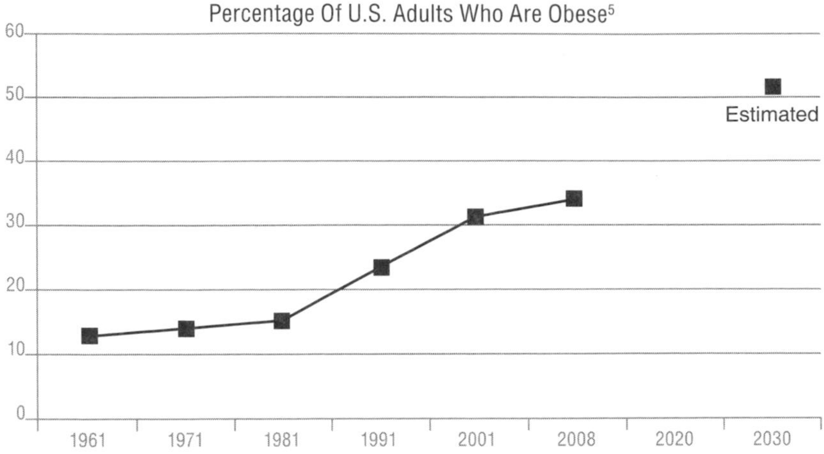

You and I may know a few people who have lost weight and kept the weight off, and we are certainly all happy for their successes. However, these small but important victories are not enough to realistically bend the obesity trend shown in this graph. I'd like to think that my books or that the wellness programs we provide to employers are having a big impact on the health of the world, but they are not. They do make a difference for some people and many are becoming healthier, but when compared to the trends of the entire U.S. population we are having very little effect. At best we may be slowing the increase, but not stopping it.

The increase in obesity shown in this graph has taken place over a period of approximately 50 years. It has taken five decades for two-thirds of the U.S. population to become overweight or obese. This is half a century of cultural changes that have ultimately resulted in nationwide weight gain. When I look at this chart and realize it has taken us 50 years to get to this point I realize that it's going to take at least 50 years to reverse this trend, and that's only if we get started right now. More than likely the obesity trend in the United States is going to get worse over the next few decades. This means that it's going to take more than 50 years before most Americans will be able to enjoy the benefits of a healthy lifestyle. You and I will be successful at creating our little islands of health, but millions of other Americans will continue to live in the unhealthy culture that surrounds us all. The obesity and diabetes epidemics in the United States will get worse before they get better. I hope I'm wrong about this prediction too, but I don't see anything in our current society that has the ability to reverse this trend.

Trend #4: Your Future Is Bright

At this point you have everything you need to improve your health and create a healthy environment that will support your efforts going forward. I've seen a lot of people attempt change, and I can usually tell how it will turn out. If you're not able to change your behaviors and alter your environment in a way that makes it easier to be healthy, not much will change. You might have a temporary improvement in your health, you might start to experience some of the benefits and you might see your health risks go down for a little while, but with time, some of you will get pulled back into our unhealthy culture and continue to live your lives the way you always have.

If, however, you are able to start taking baby steps towards creating your own island of health exciting changes will occur. Between now and six weeks from now you will change your behaviors by eating healthier and exercising more. While you may not realize it or even feel it, these changes in your behaviors will impact the physiology of your body in such a way that your blood pressure, glucose and cholesterol levels will improve. In the studies that we've published, we've seen dramatic changes in as little as six weeks. If you maintain your healthy behaviors, the great changes you've experienced at six weeks will continue to improve. Your healthy behaviors will be maintained, and your health risks will continue to improve until they reach and maintain ideal levels. When you stick with healthy behaviors, you will continue to reap all the benefits of a healthy lifestyle; you'll be able to experience the benefits for months and even years to come.[6–8]

The long-term benefits of your new healthy lifestyle are the best ones. These include extending the length of your life, improving the quality of your life and avoiding most of the common chronic diseases that afflict so many. It is these benefits that make all of your struggles and efforts to be healthy worth it.

In preparation for this book I interviewed a lot of people who had created islands of health. I asked a lot of questions and from their responses I wrote the stories you see at the end of each chapter. The last Island Native story in this book is YOUR story. You are the next Island Native to tell your story about how you were successful at transforming your life. As you can see, the following text box has some questions and blanks that I would like you to complete. When you've created your own healthy culture, complete this questionnaire so you can tell your story of how you won the battle for better health.

Island Native

It's your turn to become the next Island Native. When you've create your own culture of health answer these questions:

How did you come to find out that your health wasn't what it should be?

What caused you to want to change your lifestyle?

What have you done to eat differently?

What have you done to get more exercise?

Did you quit smoking and if so, how?

Do you have others helping you? Who? How do they help?

For many people, changing lifestyle habits is hard. How do you stay motivated to stick to it?

If you could say anything to people struggling with poor health behaviors what would you say?

References

Chapter 1:

1. Prevalence of Overweight, Obesity, and Extreme Obesity Among Adults: United States, Trends 1960–1962 Through 2007–2008, http://www.cdc.gov/nchs/data/hestat/obesity_adult_07_08/obesity_adult_07_08.htm
2. Wang Y, Beydoun MA, Liang L, Caballero B, Kumanyika SK, *Will All Americans become overweight or obese? Estimating the progression and cost of the US obesity epidemic.* Obesity 2008 Oct;16(10):2323-30. PLoS Med. 2010 Mar 23;7(3):e1000248.
3. Johnson F, Cooke L, Croker H, Wardle J, *Changing Perceptions Of Weight In Great Britain: Comparison Of Two Population Surveys.* BMJ. 2008 Jul 10;337:a494.
4. Towns N, D'Auria J, *Parental Perceptions Of Their Child's Overweight: An Integrative Review Of The Literature.* J Pediatr Nurs. 2009 Apr;24(2):115-30.
5. Duffey KJ, Popkin BM. *Energy Density, Portion Size, And Eating Occasions: Contributions To Increased Energy Intake In The United States*, 1977-2006.PLoS Med. 2011 Jun;8(6):e1001050.
6. Diliberti N, Bordi PL, Conklin MT, Roe LS, Rolls BJ.Increased portion size leads to increased energy intake in a restaurant meal. Obes Res. 2004 Mar;12(3):562-8.
7. Danaei G, Rimm EB, Oza S, Kulkarni SC, Murray CJ, Ezzati M, *The Promise Of Prevention: The Effects Of Four Preventable Risk Factors On National Life Expectancy And Life Expectancy Disparities By Race And County In The United States.* PLoS Med. 2010 Mar 23;7(3):e1000248.
8. Ezzati M, Friedman AB, Kulkarni SC, Murray CJ. *The Reversal Of Fortunes: Trends In County Mortality And Cross-County Mortality Disparities In The United States.* PLoS Med. 2008 Apr 22;5(4):e66.
9. Kulkarni SC, Levin-Rector A, Ezzati M, Murray CJ. *Falling Behind: Life Expectancy In Us Counties From 2000 To 2007 In An International Context.* Popul Health Metr. 2011 Jun 15;9(1):16.

10. Narayan KM, Boyle JP, Thompson TJ, Sorensen SW, Williamson DF, *Lifetime Risk For Diabetes Mellitus In The United States.* JAMA. 2003 Oct 8;290(14):1884-90.
11. NCHS Data Brief, *Death In The United States*, 2009, Number 64, July 2011.
12. Crimmins EM, Beltrán-Sánchez H. *Mortality And Morbidity Trends: Is There Compression Of Morbidity?* J Gerontol B Psychol Sci Soc Sci. 2011 Jan;66(1):75-86.
13. Healthy People 2000: *National Health Promotion And Disease Prevention Objectives.* Washington, D.C.: Government Printing Office, 1991. (DHHS publication no. (PHS) 91-50213.)

Chapter 2:

1. Hill A, Ward S, Deino A, Curtis G, Drake R. *Earliest Homo. Nature.* 1992 Feb 20;355(6362):719-22.
2. Levy S, et al. *The Diploid Genome Sequence Of An Individual Human.* PLoS Biol. 2007 Sep 4;5(10):e254.
3. Storck J. Teague WD. *Flour For Man's Bread, A History Of Milling.* Minneapolis: University of Minnesota Press, 1952
4. Galloway JH. 2000. Sugar. In: Kiple KF, Ornelas IKC, eds. *The Cambridge World History Of Food. Vol 1.* Cambridge: Cambridge University Press, 2000:437-49.
5. Hanover LM, White JS. *Manufacturing, Composition, And Applications Of Fructose.* Am J Clin Nutr. 1993 Nov;58(5 Suppl):724S-732S.
6. Cordain L, Eaton SB, Sebastian A, Mann N, Lindeberg S, Watkins BA, O'Keefe JH, Brand-Miller J. *Origins And Evolution Of The Western Diet: Health Implications For The 21St Century.* Am J Clin Nutr. 2005 Feb;81(2):341-54.
7. Richards MP, Pettitt PB, Trinkaus E, Smith FH, Paunović M, Karavanić I. *Neanderthal Diet At Vindija And Neanderthal Predation: The Evidence From Stable Isotopes.* Proc Natl Acad Sci U S A. 2000 Jun 20;97(13):7663-6.
8. Konner M, Eaton SB. *Paleolithic Nutrition: Twenty-Five Years Later.* Nutr Clin Pract. 2010 Dec;25(6):594-602.
9. Kidwell B. *All Grass, No Grain.* Progressive Farmer Magazine, 8 October 2002.
10. Santarelli RL, Pierre F, Corpet DE. *Processed Meat And Colorectal Cancer: A Review Of Epidemiologic And Experimental Evidence.* Nutr Cancer. 2008;60(2):131-44.
11. Salt Lake Tribune, Oct 1, 2008, http://archive.sltrib.com/article.php?id=10604809&itype=NGPSID
12. Torpy JM, Lynm C, Glass RM. JAMA patient page. *Eating Fish: Health Benefits And Risks.* JAMA. 2006 Oct 18;296(15):1926.
13. USDA http://www.usda.gov/factbook/chapter2.pdf
14. Jew S, AbuMweis SS, Jones PJ. *Evolution Of The Human Diet: Linking Our Ancestral Diet To Modern Functional Foods As A Means Of Chronic Disease Prevention.* J Med Food. 2009 Oct;12(5):925-34.
15. O'Keefe JH, Vogel R, Lavie CJ, Cordain L. *Achieving Hunter-Gatherer Fitness In The 21(St) Century: Back To The Future.* Am J Med. 2010 Dec;123(12):1082-6. Epub 2010 Sep 16.
16. Cordain L, Gotshall RW, Eaton SB, Eaton SB 3rd. *Physical Activity, Energy Expenditure And Fitness: An Evolutionary Perspective.* Int J Sports Med. 1998 Jul;19(5):328-35.

17. Panter-Brick C. *Sexual Division Of Labor: Energetic And Evolutionary Scenarios.* Am J Hum Biol. 2002 Sep-Oct;14(5):627-40.
18. Eaton SB, Eaton SB 3rd. *Paleolithic Vs. Modern Diets—Selected Pathophysiological Implications.* Eur J Nutr. 2000 Apr;39(2):67-70.
19. O'Keefe JH, Gheewala NM, O'Keefe JO. *Dietary Strategies For Improving Post-Prandial Glucose, Lipids, Inflammation, And Cardiovascular Health.* J Am Coll Cardiol. 2008 Jan 22;51(3):249-55.
20. Li C, Ford ES, McGuire LC, Mokdad AH, Little RR, Reaven GM. *Trends In Hyperinsulinemia Among Nondiabetic Adults In The US Diabetes Care.* 2006 Nov;29(11):2396-402.

Chapter 3:

1. Ayyad C, Andersen T. *Long-Term Efficacy Of Dietary Treatment Of Obesity: A Systematic Review Of Studies Published Between 1931 And 1999.* Obes Rev. 2000 Oct;1(2):113-9.
2. Sassi, F. et al. (2009), "The Obesity Epidemic: Analysis of Past and Projected Future Trends in Selected OECD Countries", *OECD Health Working Papers, No. 45,* OECD Publishing. http://dx.doi.org/10.1787/225215402672
3. Bauman A, Bull F, Chey T, Craig CL, Ainsworth BE, Sallis JF, Bowles HR, Hagstromer M, Sjostrom M, Pratt M; The IPS Group. *The International Prevalence Study On Physical Activity: Results From 20 Countries.* Int J Behav Nutr Phys Act. 2009 Mar 1;6(1):21.
4. Misra A, et al. *Consensus Dietary Guidelines For Healthy Living And Prevention Of Obesity, The Metabolic Syndrome, Diabetes, And Related Disorders In Asian Indians.* Diabetes Technol Ther. 2011 Jun;13(6):683-94.
5. Sharma S. *Assessing Diet And Lifestyle In The Canadian Arctic Inuit And Inuvialuit To Inform A Nutrition And Physical Activity Intervention Programme.* J Hum Nutr Diet. 2010 Oct;23 Suppl 1:5-17.
6. Wild S, Roglic G, Green A, Sicree R, King H. *Global Prevalence Of Diabetes: Estimates For The Year 2000 And Projections For 2030.* Diabetes Care. 2004 May;27(5):1047-53.
7. Popkin BM, Adair LS, Ng SW. *Global Nutrition Transition And The Pandemic Of Obesity In Developing Countries.* Nutr Rev. 2012 Jan;70(1):3-21.
8. Hamdan, S, *Rapid Increase Of Diabetes Strains Middle East's Health Agencies, New York Times,* January 12, 2011 available on line at: http://www.nytimes.com/2011/01/13/world/middleeast/13iht-M13CDIABET.html?_r=1
9. Torun B, Stein AD, Schroeder D, Grajeda R, Conlisk A, Rodriguez M, Mendez H, Martorell R. *Rural-To-Urban Migration And Cardiovascular Disease Risk Factors In Young Guatemalan Adults.* Int J Epidemiol. 2002 Feb;31(1):218-26.
10. Batis C, Hernandez-Barrera L, Barquera S, Rivera JA, Popkin BM. *Food Acculturation Drives Dietary Differences Among Mexicans, Mexican Americans, And Non-Hispanic Whites.* J Nutr. 2011 Oct;141(10):1898-906.
11. Lassetter JH, Callister LC. *The Impact Of Migration On The Health Of Voluntary Migrants In Western Societies.* J Transcult Nurs. 2009 Jan;20(1):93-104.
12. Goel MS, McCarthy EP, Phillips RS, Wee CC. *Obesity Among US Immigrant Subgroups By Duration Of Residence.* JAMA. 2004 Dec 15;292(23):2860-7.

13. Satia-Abouta J, Patterson RE, Neuhouser ML, Elder J. *Dietary Acculturation: Applications To Nutrition Research And Dietetics.* J Am Diet Assoc. 2002 Aug;102(8):1105-18.
14. Robertson TL, et al. *Epidemiologic Studies Of Coronary Heart Disease And Stroke In Japanese Men Living In Japan, Hawaii And California. Incidence Of Myocardial Infarction And Death From Coronary Heart Disease.* Am J Cardiol. 1977 Feb; 39(2): 239–43.
15. Oza-Frank R, Cunningham SA. *The Weight Of US Residence Among Immigrants: A Systematic Review.* Obes Rev. 2010 Apr;11(4):271-80.
16. Mulasi-Pokhriyal U, Smith C, Franzen-Castle L. *Investigating Dietary Acculturation And Intake Among US-Born And Thailand/Laos-Born Hmong-American Children Aged 9-18 Years.* Public Health Nutr. 2011 Aug 2:1-10.
17. Chiu JF, Bell AD, Herman RJ, Hill MD, Stewart JA, Cohen EA, Liau CS, Steg PG, Bhatt DL; REACH Registry Investigators. *Cardiovascular Risk Profiles And Outcomes Of Chinese Living Inside And Outside China.* Eur J Cardiovasc Prev Rehabil. 2010 Dec;17(6):668-75.
18. Singh M, Kirchengast S. *Obesity Prevalence And Nutritional Habits Among Indian Women: A Comparison Between Punjabi Women Living In India And Punjabi Migrants In Vienna, Austria.* Anthropol Anz. 2011;68(3):239-51.
19. Guendelman MD, Cheryan S, Monin B. *Fitting In But Getting Fat: Identity Threat And Dietary Choices Among U.s. Immigrant Groups.* Psychol Sci. 2011 Jul;22(7):959-67.

Chapter 4:

1. Cocores JA, Gold MS. *The Salted Food Addiction Hypothesis May Explain Overeating And The Obesity Epidemic.* Med Hypotheses. 2009 Dec;73(6):892-9.
2. Lustig RH, Schmidt LA, Brindis CD. *Public Health: The Toxic Truth About Sugar.* Nature. 2012 Feb 1;482(7383):27-29.
3. de Castro JM, Bellisle F, Dalix AM, Pearcey SM. *Palatability And Intake Relationships In Free-Living Humans. Characterization And Independence Of Influence In North Americans.* Physiol Behav. 2000 Aug-Sep;70(3-4):343-50. http://www.meatpoultry.com/News/News%20Home/Special%20Reports/2011/10/Bacons%20on%20fire.aspx
4. Brennan K, Roberts DC, Anisman H, Merali Z. *Individual Differences In Sucrose Consumption In The Rat: Motivational And Neurochemical Correlates Of Hedonia.* Psychopharmacology (Berl). 2001 Sep;157(3):269-76.
5. Ward SJ, Dykstra LA. *The Role Of CB1 Receptors In Sweet Versus Fat Reinforcement: Effect Of CB1 Receptor Deletion, CB1 Receptor Antagonism (Sr141716a) And CB1 Receptor Agonism (Cp-55940).* Behav Pharmacol. 2005 Sep;16(5-6):381-8.
6. Ward SJ, Rosenberg M, Dykstra LA, Walker EA. The CB1 antagonist rimonabant (SR141716) blocks cue-induced reinstatement of cocaine seeking and other context and extinction phenomena predictive of relapse. *Drug Alcohol Depend.* 2009 Dec 1;105(3):248-55.
7. Ifland JR, Preuss HG, Marcus MT, Rourke KM, Taylor WC, Burau K, Jacobs

WS, Kadish W, Manso G. *Refined Food Addiction: A Classic Substance Use Disorder.* Med Hypotheses. 2009 May;72(5):518-26.

8. Briefel RR, Johnson CL. *Secular Trends In Dietary Intake In The United States.* Annu Rev Nutr. 2004;24:401-431
9. Centers for Disease Control and Prevention (CDC) *Sodium Intake Among Adults - United States, 2005-2006.* MMWR Morb Mortal Wkly Rep. 2010 Jun 25;59(24):746-9.
10. Sacks FM, Svetkey LP, Vollmer WM, Appel LJ, Bray GA, Harsha D, Obarzanek E, Conlin PR, Miller ER 3rd, Simons-Morton DG, Karanja N, Lin PH; *DASH-Sodium Collaborative Research Group. Effects On Blood Pressure Of Reduced Dietary Sodium And The Dietary Approaches To Stop Hypertension (DASH) Diet.* DASH-Sodium Collaborative Research Group. N Engl J Med. 2001 Jan 4;344(1):3-10.

Chapter 5:

1. Centers for Disease Control and Prevention. Annual Smoking-Attributable Mortality, Years of Potential Life Lost, and Productivity Losses—United States, 1995–1999. *Morbidity And Mortality Weekly Report* 2002;51(14):300–3.
2. Centers for Disease Control and Prevention. Smoking-Attributable Mortality, Years of Potential Life Lost, and Productivity Losses—United States, 2000–2004. *Morbidity And Mortality Weekly Report* 2008;57(45):1226–8.
World Health Organization. *WHO Report On The Global Tobacco Epidemic,* 2009. Geneva: World Health Organization, 2008.
3. Chaloupka, FJ, "Macro-Social Influences: The Effects of Prices and Tobacco Control Policies on the Demand for Tobacco Products," *Nicotine And Tobacco Research* 1(Suppl 1):S105-9, 1999.
4. Karppanen H, Mervaala E. *Sodium Intake And Hypertension.* Prog Cardiovasc Dis. 2006;49:59-75.
5. Ludwig DS, Peterson KE, Gortmaker SL. *Relation Between Consumption Of Sugar-Sweetened Drinks And Childhood Obesity: A Prospective, Observational Analysis.* Lancet. 2001;357:505-508.
6. Duffey KJ, Popkin BM. *Energy Density, Portion Size, And Eating Occasions: Contributions To Increased Energy Intake In The United States,* 1977-2006. PLoS Med. 2011 Jun;8(6):e1001050.
7. USDA, *Diet Quality And Food Consumption,* 2001, http://www.ers.usda.gov/Briefing/DietQuality/FAFH.htm
8. Todd J, Mancino L, Lin B. *The Impact Of Food Away From Home On Adult Diet Quality.* Economic Research Report No. (ERR-90) 24 pp, February 2010. http://www.ers.usda.gov/Publications/ERR90/ERR90_ReportSummary.pdf
9. USDA Agriculture Fact Book 2001-2002, Chapter 2. *Profiling Food Consumption In America,* 2001 www.usda.gov/factbook/
10. Jew S, AbuMweis SS, Jones PJ. *Evolution Of The Human Diet: Linking Our Ancestral Diet To Modern Functional Foods As A Means Of Chronic Disease Prevention.* J Med Food. 2009 Oct;12(5):925-34.
11. Poti JM, Popkin BM. *Trends In Energy Intake Among US Children By Eating Location And*

Food Source, 1977-2006. J Am Diet Assoc. 2011 Aug;111(8):1156-64.

12. McCrory MA, Fuss PJ, Hays NP, Vinken AG, Greenberg AS, Roberts SB. *Overeating In America: Association Between Restaurant Food Consumption And Body Fatness In Healthy Adult Men And Women Ages 19 To 80.* Obes Res. 1999;7:564-571.
13. Bes-Rastrollo M, van Dam RM, Martinez-Gonzalez MA, Li TY, Sampson LL, Hu FB. *Prospective Study Of Dietary Energy Density And Weight Gain In Women.* Am J Clin Nutr. 2008 Sep;88(3):769-77.
14. Savage JS, Marini M, Birch LL. *Dietary Energy Density Predicts Women's Weight Change Over 6 Years.* Am J Clin Nutr. 2008 Sep;88(3):677-84.
15. Rolls BJ, Kim S, Fedoroff IC. *Effects Of Drinks Sweetened With Sucrose Or Aspartame On Hunger, Thirst And Food Intake In Men.* Physiol Behav. 1990;48:19-26.
16. Ludwig DS, Peterson KE, Gortmaker SL. *Relation Between Consumption Of Sugar-Sweetened Drinks And Childhood Obesity: A Prospective, Observational Analysis.* Lancet. 2001;357:505-508.
17. Nielsen SJ, Popkin BM. *Patterns And Trends In Food Portion Sizes,* 1977-1998. JAMA. 2003 Jan 22-29;289(4):450-3.
18. Schwartz J, Byrd-Bredbenner C. *Portion Distortion: Typical Portion Sizes Selected By Young Adults.* J Am Diet Assoc. 2006 Sep;106(9):1412-8.
19. Rolls BJ, Roe LS, Meengs JS. *Larger Portion Sizes Lead To A Sustained Increase In Energy Intake Over Two Days.* J Am Diet Assoc. 2006 Apr;106(4):543-9.
20. Rolls BJ, Morris EL, Roe LS. *Portion Size Of Food Affects Energy Intake In Normal-Weight And Overweight Men And Women.* Am J Clin Nutr. 2002;76:1207-1213.
21. Steenhuis IH, Leeuwis FH, Vermeer WM. *Small, Medium, Large Or Supersize: Trends In Food Portion Sizes In The Netherlands* Public Health Nutr. 2010 Jun;13(6):852-7.

Chapter 6:

1. Ely JJ, Zavaskis T, Wilson SL. *Diabetes And Stress: An Anthropological Review For Study Of Modernizing Populations In The US-Mexico Border Region Rural Remote Health.* 2011;11(3):1758.
2. Schulz LO, Bennett PH, Ravussin E, Kidd JR, Kidd KK, Esparza J, Valencia ME. *Effects Of Traditional And Western Environments On Prevalence Of Type 2 Diabetes In Pima Indians In Mexico And The US.* Diabetes Care. 2006 Aug;29(8):1866-71.
3. Kung HC, Hoyert DL, Xu JQ, Murphy SL. Deaths: final data for 2005. *National Vital Statistics Reports* 2008;56(10). Available from: http://www.cdc.gov/nchs/data/nvsr/nvsr56/nvsr56_10.pdf
4. Noren, M. *Critical Mass Crisis: Child Obesity,* ESPN commentary, Mar 26, 2009 on the web at: http://sports.espn.go.com/espn/otl/news/story?id=4015831
5. Kaiser Family Foundation, *Daily Media Use Among Children And Teens Up Dramatically From Five Years Ago*, Jan 20, 2010, on line at: http://www.kff.org/entmedia/entmedia012010nr.cfm
6. Rideout V. Vandewater E. Wartella E. *Zero To Six Electronic Media In The Lives Of*

Infants, Toddlers, And Preschoolers, Fall 2003, Kaiser Family Foundation.

7. Sandercock GR, Ogunleye AA. *Screen Time And Passive School Travel As Independent Predictors Of Cardiorespiratory Fitness In Youth.* Prev Med. 2012 May 1;54(5):319-22.
8. BRFSS, *Behavior Risk Factor Surveillance System*, on the web at: http://www.cdc.gov/brfss/
9. Nikander R, Sievänen H, Heinonen A, Daly RM, Uusi-Rasi K, Kannus P. *Targeted Exercise Against Osteoporosis: A Systematic Review And Meta-Analysis For Optimising Bone Strength Throughout Life.* Eura Medicophys. 2004 Sep;40(3):199-209.
10. Manson JE, Hu FB, Rich-Edwards JW, Colditz GA, Stampfer MJ, Willett WC, Speizer FE, Hennekens CH. *A Prospective Study Of Walking As Compared With Vigorous Exercise In The Prevention Of Coronary Heart Disease In Women.* N Engl J Med. 1999 Aug 26;341(9):650-8.
11. Oldridge NB. *Compliance And Exercise In Primary And Secondary Prevention Of Coronary Heart Disease: A Review.* Prev Med. 1982 Jan;11(1):56-70
12. Anzuini F, Battistella A, Izzotti A. *Physical Activity And Cancer Prevention: A Review Of Current Evidence And Biological Mechanisms.* J Prev Med Hyg. 2011 Dec;52(4):174-80.
13. Hu FB, Manson JE, Stampfer MJ, Colditz G, Liu S, Solomon CG, Willett WC. *Diet, Lifestyle, And The Risk Of Type 2 Diabetes Mellitus In Women.* N Engl J Med. 2001 Sep 13;345(11):790-7.
14. Kubitz KA, Landers DM, Petruzzello SJ, Han M. *The Effects Of Acute And Chronic Exercise On Sleep. A Meta-Analytic Review.* Sports Med. 1996 Apr;21(4):277-91.
15. Lamina S, Agbanusi E, Nwacha RC. *Effects Of Aerobic Exercise In The Management Of Erectile Dysfunction: A Meta Analysis Study On Randomized Controlled Trials.* Ethiop J Health Sci. 2011 Nov;21(3):195-201.
16. Lee JH, Ngengwe R, Jones P, Tang F, O'Keefe JH. *Erectile Dysfunction As A Coronary Artery Disease Risk Equivalent.* J Nucl Cardiol. 2008 Nov-Dec;15(6):800-3.
17. Meldrum DR, Gambone JC, Morris MA, Meldrum DA, Esposito K, Ignarro LJ. *The Link Between Erectile And Cardiovascular Health: The Canary In The Coal Mine.* Am J Cardiol. 2011 Aug 15;108(4):599-606.
18. Norton MC, Dew J, Smith H, Fauth E, Piercy KW, Breitner JC, Tschanz J, Wengreen H, Welsh-Bohmer K; Cache County Investigators. *Lifestyle Behavior Pattern Is Associated With Different Levels Of Risk For Incident Dementia And Alzheimer's Disease: The Cache County Study.* J Am Geriatr Soc. 2012 Mar;60(3):405-12.
19. Aldana SG, Barlow M, Smith R, Yanowitz FG, Adams T, Loveday L, Arbuckle J, LaMonte MJ. *The Diabetes Prevention Program: A Worksite Experience* AAOHN J. 2005 Nov;53(11):499-505; quiz 506-7.
20. Aldana S, Barlow M, Smith R, Yanowitz F, Adams T, Loveday L, Merrill RM. *A Worksite Diabetes Prevention Program: Two-Year Impact On Employee Health.* AAOHN J. 2006 Sep;54(9):389-95.
21. Fontaine KR, Redden DT, Wang C, Westfall AO, Allison DB. *Years Of Life Lost Due To Obesity.* JAMA. 2003 Jan 8;289(2):187-93. Fraser GE, Shavlik DJ. *Ten Years Of Life: Is It A Matter Of Choice?* Arch Intern Med. 2001 Jul 9;161(13):1645-52.

22. Garber CE, Blissmer B, Deschenes MR, Franklin BA, Lamonte MJ, Lee IM, Nieman DC, Swain DP; American College of Sports Medicine. *American College Of Sports Medicine Position Stand.* Quantity and quality of exercise for developing and maintaining cardiorespiratory, musculoskeletal, and neuromotor fitness in apparently healthy adults: guidance for prescribing exercise. Med Sci Sports Exerc. 2011 Jul;43(7):1334-59.
23. Merrill RM, Anderson A, Thygerson SM. *Effectiveness Of A Worksite Wellness Program On Health Behaviors And Personal Health.* J Occup Environ Med. 2011 Sep;53(9):1008-12.

Chapter 7:

1. Wang Y, Beydoun MA, Liang L, Caballero B, Kumanyika SK, *Will All Americans Become Overweight Or Obese? Estimating The Progression And Cost Of The US Obesity Epidemic.* Obesity 2008 Oct;16(10):2323-30.
2. Luke 16:13 "No servant can serve two masters: for either he will hate the one, and love the other; or else he will hold to the one, and despise the other." From the Book of Luke in the New Testament.
3. New York Times, *While Warning About Fat, US Pushes Cheese Sales*, Nov 6, 2010, Found on the web at: http://www.nytimes.com/2010/11/07/us/07fat.html?pagewanted=2&_r=2
4. Lanou AJ, Barnard ND. *Dairy And Weight Loss Hypothesis: An Evaluation Of The Clinical Trials.* Nutr Rev. 2008 May;66(5):272-9.
5. FDA, *US Food And Drug Administration's Health And Diet Survey 2008*, on the web at: http://www.fda.gov/Food/ScienceResearch/ResearchAreas/ConsumerResearch/ucm193895.htm
6. Swartz JJ, Braxton D, Viera AJ. *Calorie Menu Labeling On Quick-Service Restaurant Menus: An Updated Systematic Review Of The Literature.* Int J Behav Nutr Phys Act. 2011 Dec 8;8:135.
7. Dumanovsky T, Huang CY, Nonas CA, Matte TD, Bassett MT, Silver LD. *Changes In Energy Content Of Lunchtime Purchases From Fast Food Restaurants After Introduction Of Calorie Labeling: Cross Sectional Customer Surveys.* BMJ. 2011 Jul 26;343:d4464.
8. Ollberding NJ, Wolf RL, Contento I. *Food Label Use And Its Relation To Dietary Intake Among US Adults.* J Am Diet Assoc. 2010 Aug;110(8):1233-7.
9. Brownell KD, Koplan JP. *Front-Of-Package Nutrition Labeling—An Abuse Of Trust By The Food Industry?* N Engl J Med. 2011 Jun 23;364(25):2373-5.
10. Sharma LL, Teret SP, Brownell KD. *The Food Industry And Self-Regulation: Standards To Promote Success And To Avoid Public Health Failures.* Am J Public Health 2010;100:240-246.

Chapter 8:

1. Stokols D. *Translating Social Ecological Theory Into Guidelines For Community Health Promotion.* Am J Health Promot. 1996 Mar-Apr;10(4):282-298.
2. Do R, Xie C, Zhang X, Männistö S, Harald K, Islam S, Bailey SD, Rangarajan S, McQueen MJ, Diaz R, Lisheng L, Wang X, Silander K, Peltonen L, Yusuf S, Salomaa V, Engert JC, Anand SS; INTERHEART investigators. *The Effect Of On Cardiovascular Disease May Be Modified By Dietary Intake: Evidence From A Case/Control And A Prospective Study.* PLoS Med. 2011 Oct;8(10).

3. Moskin J. *Chef Has Diabetes,* and *Some Say 'I Told You So',* New York Times, Jan 17, 2012.
4. Executive summary of the third report on the *National Cholesterol Education Program (NCEP)* expert panel on detection, evaluation, and treatment of high blood cholesterol in adults (adult treatment panel III). JAMA 285:2486–97. 2001.
5. Ervin RB. *Prevalence Of Metabolic Syndrome Among Adults 20 Years Of Age And Over, By Sex, Age, Race And Ethnicity, And Body Mass Index: United States,* 2003-2006. Natl Health Stat Report. 2009 May 5;(13):1-7.
6. Stampfer MJ, Hu FB, Manson JE, Rimm EB, Willett WC. *Primary Prevention Of Coronary Heart Disease In Women Through Diet And Lifestyle.* N Engl J Med 2000 Jul 6;343(1):16–22.
7. Platz EA, Willett WC, Colditz GA, Rimm EB, Spiegelman D, Giovannucci E. *Proportion Of Colon Cancer Risk That Might Be Preventable In A Cohort Of Middle-Aged US Men.* Cancer Causes Control 2000 Aug;11(7):579–88.
8. Hu FB, Manson JE, Stampfer MJ, Colditz G, Liu S, Solomon CG, Willett WC. *Diet, Lifestyle, And The Risk Of Type 2 Diabetes Mellitus In Women.* N Engl J Med 2001 Sep 13;345(11):790–7.
9. American College of Preventive Medicine, *Lifestyle Medicine—Evidence Review,* June 30, 2009 on the web at: http://www.acpm.org/resource/resmgr/lmi-files/lifestylemedicine-literature.pdf
10. Daviglus ML, Stamler J, Pirzada A, Yan LL, Garside DB, Liu K, Wang R, Dyer AR, Lloyd-Jones DM, Greenland P. *Favorable Cardiovascular Risk Profile In Young Women And Long-Term Risk Of Cardiovascular And All-Cause Mortality.* JAMA. 2004;292:1588 –1592.
11. Stamler J, Stamler R, Neaton JD, Wentworth D, Daviglus ML, Garside D, Dyer AR, Liu K, Greenland P. *Low Risk-Factor Profile And Long-Term Cardiovascular And Noncardiovascular Mortality And Life Expectancy: Findings For 5 Large Cohorts Of Young Adult And Middle-Aged Men And Women.* JAMA. 1999;282:2012–2018.
12. Daviglus ML, Liu K, Pirzada A, Yan LL, Garside DB, Feinglass J, Guralnik JM, Greenland P, Stamler J. *Favorable Cardiovascular Risk Profile In Middle Age And Health-Related Quality Of Life In Older Age.* Arch Intern Med. 2003;163:2460 –2468.
13. Daviglus ML, Liu K, Greenland P, Dyer AR, Garside DB, Manheim L, Lowe LP, Rodin M, Lubitz J, Stamler J. *Benefit Of A Favorable Cardiovascular Risk-Factor Profile In Middle Age With Respect To Medicare Costs.* N Engl J Med. 1998;339:1122–1129.
14. Kvaavik E, Batty GD, Ursin G, Huxley R, Gale CR. *Influence Of Individual And Combined Health Behaviors On Total And Cause-Specific Mortality In Men And Women. The United Kingdom Health And Lifestyle Survey.* Arch Intern Med. 2010 Apr 26;170(8):711-8.
15. Khaw KT, Wareham N, Bingham S, Welch A, Luben R, Day N. *Combined Impact Of Health Behaviours And Mortality In Men And Women: The EPIC-Norfolk Prospective Population Study.* PLoS Med. 2008 Jan 8;5(1):e12.
16. Mozaffarian D, Kamineni A, Carnethon M, Djoussé L, Mukamal KJ, Siscovick

D. *Lifestyle Risk Factors And New-Onset Diabetes Mellitus In Older Adults: The Cardiovascular Health Study.* Arch Intern Med. 2009 Apr 27;169(8):798-807.

17. Rowley KG, Daniel M, Skinner K, Skinner M, White GA, O'Dea K. *Effectiveness Of A Community-Directed 'Healthy Lifestyle' Program In A Remote Australian Aboriginal Community.* Aust N Z J Public Health. 2000 Apr;24(2):136-44.
18. Poulain M, Pes GM, Grasland C, Carru C, Ferrucci L, Baggio G, Franceschi C, Deiana L. *Identification Of A Geographic Area Characterized By Extreme Longevity In The Sardinia Island: The Akea Study.* Exp Gerontol. 2004 Sep;39(9):1423-9.
19. Willcox DC, Willcox BJ, Hsueh WC, Suzuki M. *Genetic Determinants Of Exceptional Human Longevity: Insights From The Okinawa Centenarian Study.* Age (Dordr). 2006 Dec;28(4):313-32.
20. Perls T, Terry D. *Understanding The Determinants Of Exceptional Longevity.* Ann Intern Med. 2003 Sep 2;139(5 Pt 2):445-450.
21. Fraser, G. Diet, *Life Expectancy, And Chronic Disease: Studies Of Seventh-Day Adventists And Other Vegetarians*, Oxford University Press, 2003.
22. Kent LM, Worsley A. *Does The Prescriptive Lifestyle Of Seventh-Day Adventists Provide 'Immunity' From The Secular Effects Of Changes In BMI?* Public Health Nutr. 2009 Apr;12(4):472-80.
23. Fraser GE. *Diet As Primordial Prevention In Seventh-Day Adventists.* Prev Med. 1999 Dec;29(6 Pt 2):S18-23.
24. Jönsson T, Ahrén B, Pacini G, Sundler F, Wierup N, Steen S, Sjöberg T, Ugander M, Frostegård J, Göransson L, Lindeberg S. *A Paleolithic Diet Confers Higher Insulin Sensitivity, Lower C-Reactive Protein And Lower Blood Pressure Than A Cereal-Based Diet In Domestic Pigs.* Nutr Metab (Lond). 2006 Nov 2;3:39.
25. Franco M, Orduñez P, Caballero B, et al. *Impact Of Energy Intake, Physical Activity, And Population-Wide Weight Loss On Cardiovascular Disease And Diabetes Mortality In Cuba*, 1980-2005. Am J Epidem 2007;15:1374-80.
26. Aldana SG, Greenlaw RL, Diehl HA, Salberg A, Merrill RM, Ohmine S, Thomas C. *The Behavioral And Clinical Effects Of Therapeutic Lifestyle Change On Middle-Aged Adults.* Prev Chronic Dis. 2006 Jan;3(1):A05.
27. Aldana SG, Greenlaw RL, Diehl HA, Salberg A, Merrill RM, Ohmine S. *The Effects Of A Worksite Chronic Disease Prevention Program.* J Occup Environ Med. 2005 Jun;47(6):558-64.
28. Aldana SG, Greenlaw RL, Diehl HA, Salberg A, Merrill RM, Ohmine S, Thomas C. *Effects Of An Intensive Diet And Physical Activity Modification Program On The Health Risks Of Adults.* J Am Diet Assoc. 2005;105(3):371-81.

Chapter 9:

1. Zhou X, Nonnemaker J, Sherrill B, Gilsenan AW, Coste F, West R. *Attempts To Quit Smoking And Relapse: Factors Associated With Success Or Failure From The ATTEMPT Cohort Study.* Addict Behav. 2009 Apr;34(4):365-73.

2. O'Donnell MP. *A Simple Framework To Describe What Works Best: Improving Awareness, Enhancing Motivation, Building Skills, And Providing Opportunity.* Am J Health Promot. 2005 Sep-Oct;20(1):suppl 1-7.
3. Clements-Thompson M, Klesges RC, Haddock K, Lando H, Talcott W. *Relationships Between Stages Of Change In Cigarette Smokers And Healthy Lifestyle Behaviors In A Population Of Young Military Personnel During Forced Smoking Abstinence.* J Consult Clin Psychol. 1998 Dec;66(6):1005-11.
4. Klesges RC, Haddock CK, Lando H, Talcott GW. *Efficacy Of Forced Smoking Cessation And An Adjunctive Behavioral Treatment On Long-Term Smoking Rates.* J Consult Clin Psychol. 1999 Dec;67(6):952-8.
5. Prochaska, J. Personal communication with Dr. James Prochaska, Director of the Cancer Prevention Research Center, University of Rhode Island, March, 2012.

Chapter 10:

1. Lecheminant JD, Merrill RM. *Improved Health Behaviors Persist Over Two Years For Employees In A Worksite Wellness Program.* Popul Health Manag. 2012 Oct;15(5):261-6.
2. Maurer, R. *One Small Step Can Change Your Life: The Kaizen Way,* 2004, Workman Publishing Company.
3. Ogden LG, Stroebele N, Wyatt HR, Catenacci VA, Peters JC, Stuht J, Wing RR, Hill JO., *Cluster Analysis Of The National Weight Control Registry To Identify Distinct Subgroups Maintaining Successful Weight Loss.* Obesity (Silver Spring). 2012 Apr 3.
4. Heath GW, Parra DC, Sarmiento OL, Andersen LB, Owen N, Goenka S, Montes F, Brownson RC; Lancet Physical Activity Series Working Group. *Evidence-Based Intervention In Physical Activity: Lessons From Around The World.* Lancet. 2012 Jul 21;380(9838):272-81.
5. Drewnowski A, Specter SE. *Poverty And Obesity: The Role Of Energy Density And Energy Costs.* Am J Clin Nutr. 2004 Jan;79(1):6-16.
6. Hruschka DJ. *Do Economic Constraints On Food Choice Make People Fat? A Critical Review Of Two Hypotheses For The Poverty-Obesity Paradox.* Am J Hum Biol. 2012 May-Jun;24(3):277-85.
7. Monsivais P, Aggarwal A, Drewnowski A. *Following Federal Guidelines To Increase Nutrient Consumption May Lead To Higher Food Costs For Consumers.* Health Aff (Millwood). 2011 Aug;30(8):1471-7.

Chapter 11:

1. Stokols D. *Translating Social Ecological Theory Into Guidelines For Community Health Promotion.* Am J Health Promot. 1996;10:282-298.
2. Wilson SE. *The Health Capital Of Families: An Investigation Of The Inter-Spousal Correlation In Health Status.* Soc Sci Med. 2002 Oct;55(7):1157-72.
3. Falba TA, Sindelar JL. *Spousal Concordance In Health Behavior Change.* Health Serv Res. 2008 Feb;43(1 Pt 1):96-116.
4. Homish GG, Leonard KE. *Spousal Influence On General Health Behaviors In A Community Sample.* Am J Health Behav. 2008 Nov-Dec;32(6):754-63.

5. Wansink B. *Nutritional Gatekeepers And The 72% Solution.* JADA. 2006 Sep;106(9):1324–1327
6. Christakis NA, Fowler JH. *The Spread Of Obesity In A Large Social Network Over 32 Years.* N Engl J Med. 2007 Jul 26;357(4):370-9.
7. Wansink B, Painter JE, Lee YK. *The Office Candy Dish: Proximity's Influence On Estimated And Actual Consumption.* Int J Obes (Lond). 2006 May;30(5):871-5.
8. Grynbaum M, *Health Panel Approves Restriction On Sale Of Large Sugary Drinks.* NY Times, Sept 13, 2012.

Chapter 12:

1. Executive Office of the President of the United States. *Solving The Problem Of Childhood Obesity Within A Generation: White House Task Force On Childhood Obesity Report To The President* [2010] OCLC Number: (OCoLC)640128347 on the web at: http://www.letsmove.gov/sites/letsmove.gov/files/TaskForce_on_Childhood_Obesity_May2010_FullReport.pdf
2. Romon M, Lommez A, Tafflet M, et al. *Downward Trends In The Prevalence Of Childhood Overweight In The Setting Of 12-Year School- And Community-Based Programmes.* Public Health Nutr 2008;12:1-8.
3. Kaiser Family Foundation and Health Research and Educational Trust. *Employer Health Benefits 2012 Annual Survey.* September 2012.
4. Centers for Medicare and Medicaid Services, Office of the Actuary, National Health Statistics Group, National Health Care Expenditures Data, January 2012.
5. *Prevalence of Overweight, Obesity, and Extreme Obesity Among Adults: United States, Trends 1960–1962 Through 2007–2008,* http://www.cdc.gov/nchs/data/hestat/obesity_adult_07_08/obesity_adult_07_08.htm
6. Aldana SG, Greenlaw RL, Diehl HA, Salberg A, Merrill RM, Ohmine S, Thomas C. *The Behavioral And Clinical Effects Of Therapeutic Lifestyle Change On Middle-Aged Adults.* Prev Chronic Dis. 2006 Jan;3(1):A05.
7. Aldana SG, Greenlaw RL, Diehl HA, Salberg A, Merrill RM, Ohmine S. *The Effects Of A Worksite Chronic Disease Prevention Program.* J Occup Environ Med. 2005 Jun;47(6):558-64.
8. Aldana SG, Greenlaw RL, Diehl HA, Salberg A, Merrill RM, Ohmine S, Thomas C. *Effects Of An Intensive Diet And Physical Activity Modification Program On The Health Risks Of Adults.* J Am Diet Assoc. 2005;105(3):371-81.

Index

E

F

G

H

I

J

K

L

M

Notes

Notes